GREG WILSON

HEALTH
4EVER

Health4Ever

Your Personal Guide to Health and Wellbeing

Greg Wilson

Health4Ever
Your Personal Guide to Health and Wellbeing

Copyright © 2023 by Greg Wilson

Paperback ISBN: 978-1-63812-901-1
Ebook ISBN: 978-1-63812-902-8

All rights reserved. No part in this book may be produced and transmitted in any form or by any means, electronic, or mechanical, including photocopying, recording, or by any information storage and retrieval system, without permission in writing from the copyright owner.

The views expressed in this work are solely those of the author and do not necessarily reflect the views of the publisher hereby disclaims any responsibility for them.

Published by Pen Culture Solutions   02/09/2023

Pen Culture Solutions
1-888-727-7204 (USA)
1-800-950-458 (Australia)
support@penculturesolutions.com

Health4ever
Your Personal Guide to Health and Wellbeing
2nd Edition

To my family; Jacinta my wife, our two boys Benjamin and Jacob.
To my brother Mark for always supporting me and to my
brother Ashley for prompting me to write this book.
I am grateful to you all!

Contents

Forward 5
Preface 7
Introduction 11
ADDENDUM..15

Section I
Concise Health Reference
A to Z Health Reference..18
Low Acid Diet plan 131
Diet and Personal Health 134
Basic Back Care...140

Section II
Living Happier
Better relationships?...150
Guiding Children...154
Communication...156
Control and Power 158
Keeping Ourselves on Track..160
Getting ahead in the world..163
Problem Solving 164
Organs of the body and related emotions. 165
Depression 166
Relaxation and Music..168
REFERENCES:..169
Summary 170
Conclusion 173
About the Author 177

Forward

Good nutritious food and clean drinking water are the main-stays of health. Unfortunately, commercialism, greed and lifestyle have largely corrupted our food supplies and the things we eat. Being aware of what foods you put into your body will bring balance to yourself and ultimately the planet. Health is a combination of factors including diet and lifestyle, a happy state of *Being* and a reduction in stress. When we balance these pillars of health we naturally drift toward happiness and can achieve our full potential in life.

The physical food that we eat also contains an implicit vibration from seed to plant to harvest to store and finally onto your plate. Every stage that food goes through affects its quality. When consuming it, that vibration is going into your body. So bless your food! Be grateful for everything.

This book will assist you on that road to true and lasting health. We stand on the pinnacle of a golden age with incredible discoveries happening now and awaiting us all on this beautiful blue planet. Science and the ancient wisdoms merge before our very eyes. Yet our bodies never needed proof for they have always known. Eat foods grown naturally and drink pure water.

Gregory Wilson has a wealth of wisdom on organics, natural eating, bodily processes and quantum biological effects. All you need to attain a healthy state of being, all contained in a concise easy reference. Simplistic, but in-depth techniques to achieve happiness through correct living coupled with insightful knowledge on what to eat and what to

avoid. Reading this wonderful book will change your life for the better and open your eyes to a whole new way of looking at food.
Ashley Wilson.

(A forward by Dorothea Saaghy)

Greg Wilson, a friend of many years, has researched the subject of health through right living, good food, physical, mental and spiritual activity very thoroughly.

To help others with his profound knowledge is a true passion. His enthusiasm shines through the words and will kindle and enrich the awareness in the reader: Transmitting energy through words is a form of healing.

So, read the book, follow the advice and explanations, take action and you will be on the way to lasting health.

And what better dwelling place, for mind and spirit, than a healthy happy body!
Dorothea Saaghy.

Preface

The concept of writing this book was borne for the reason that we seem to be mis-guided with regards to good health.

If someone develops an illness or requires hospitalization then once they recover they do not receive sound, yet basic health advice. They are left in the dark as to what to do. We all need to take a little more responsibility of our own health, that does not require drastic changes nor enrolling in a health course of some sought.

Herein lies some basic, concise information on common health complaints that we all can relate to and understand. It is through this understanding that we can exercise choice whether to act on our own health! I hope this book helps us all to look into our health.

<u>It is no good taking cough medicine every time we catch a cold. What we should be doing is addressing the cause of why we catch so many colds.</u>

This book is designed to help you be happy and healthy. It is a concise health reference for common ailments that also includes many fascinating facts on health. In section II the book is about how to live happier and offers some interesting thoughts, ideas and insights into life, and, how to get the best out of your relationships with others. We all would like to get along better in the world; just think of the benefits, globally, when we come closer to achieving this.

I have set the book out to offer concise, (not long winded), information. Once we are better informed, with regards to our health, then we can make better decisions. I know some people are not interested in health nor looking after oneself, but, once a debilitating illness takes hold then they want help straight away. I feel it is advantageous to know more than to know less when it comes to our personal health.

I have experienced health problems too. I was about to undergo surgery on a nerve problem in my hand. After researching my complaint further, I then received several treatments from an acupuncturist and masseur. Two weeks later I cancelled the surgery.

Now there are times when we need to take advice first hand, I understand that, as there could be life threatening consequences if not heeded. With the example I mentioned above, I researched and acquired specific information that enabled me to fully understand my health concern and make an informed decision.

I took it upon myself to continue researching matters of health a couple of decades ago and to this day I am convinced that we can improve our health; we can make better decisions in life when we are better informed. I hope you will get a great deal of sound ideas from this book and use some of them for your family and yourself.

For many years now I have seen how our health is declining ever so slowly despite wonderful advancements in medicine. I feel we are misguided and not truly informed of our health and how we can make a difference to achieve Health 4 Ever. Ignorance is not a virtue! We have been misguided somewhat. We have been coerced into believing that we cannot overcome modern day illnesses. Maybe through this coercion we start to accept this fact. Well, I can tell you now, quite categorically, that if you pay attention to correct nutrition, lifestyle and psychological health you can make a difference.

There are groups of people throughout the world that do not get modern day illnesses. For example; arthritis, blood diseases, cholesterol problems—even cancer. You have to ask the question, "why?"

The media, some food companies, the medical and pharmaceutical industries play such a vital role in our health and, therefore, have a persuasive and influential outcome on our thoughts and beliefs with regards to <u>our</u> health: Maybe they should be a little more responsible with their influence on our health. I might add that most all health professionals do the right thing and have a vested interest in our better health – I cannot over-emphasize this, without our dedicated doctors and nurses we would be struggling with illnesses. I hold them in high regards.

However, de-natured foods, <u>even though we may think we are eating right</u>, are having a major impact on our lives. The doctors and hospitals do not have the time, nor the training, to put into guiding us with correct nutrition and lifestyle choices.

As mentioned, I personally, experienced health problems. Having tried the orthodox approaches without much success. I started to explore other possibilities of health improvement. That is when I saw great value in correct nutrition, lifestyle and other health factors. In the book I have further personal examples of health improvement.

This leads on to the reason why I wrote this book; to inform, to educate, to motivate us all to help take responsibility and control of our own health so that our future life is not so debilitating, nor dependent on the medical and hospital fraternity. If you work with some of the ideas and thoughts of true health contained herein I passionately know you can address modern health illnesses.

Once given better information regarding our personal health then we can decide to do something about it, or, we can choose to continue down the existing path – it is a matter of choice.

Health 4 Ever

Introduction

The aim of this book is to combine principles on living happier along with (better) understanding of health and illnesses: Health and happiness are intrinsically linked in profound ways! **You cannot have one without the other – it just won't work in life!**

Are modern day illnesses and diseases addressable? Yes, they are…

Being better informed about our health enables us to take action. One problem I see is that we tend to expect our doctors and nurses to have all the solutions to our health.

We often overlook our nutrition plan in daily life so this book is designed to give some succinct and informative ideas on attaining health forever.

> **Meal preparation hints, tests that you can perform at home or through your doctor, fingernail patterns that show signs of pending health issues, etc. These and many more interesting, and often unheard of facts you will find in the book that can help pre-warn of future health problems.**

There is a huge misconception that we cannot improve our health, especially our modern-day diseases —arthritis and cancers, to name only two. Well, we can improve our health! A lot of our physical illnesses are centered around three things;
1. Poor nutritional foods and overloading with artificial foods
2. Poor digestion of these foods
3. A weak immune system

If you elect to ignore good health then that is your choice. However, a little understanding and some minor adjustments to your lifestyle will help to add years of pain free health to your life. Here I offer you the chance to gain better information on health and how this affects us. I lay it out on the table so to speak, so you can make a decision without the influence of commercialism, the media and other related groups that have their own agenda – not your health in mind.

In section 1 you will find a concise health reference that you can look up to find fascinating information on common health ailments and many other interesting facts relating to health and nutrition.

In section II I look at ways to live a happier life, striving for wellbeing of the mind. I know that in our modern, fast paced world, things may not always work out as we would like. However, there are some basic things we can pay attention to that can have a very positive impact on our relationships with others, more importantly, with ourselves! I have observed interactions of people going about their daily activities and have noticed that we all can do with a few pointers to keep us on track, and to make our relationships, more importantly, with others a better experience for all.

This A to Z reference quickly gives you information that we all can relate to – concise, accurate, easy-to-understand! I have taken the liberty to exclude some detailed explanations. We do not necessarily need to know all the facts. The content of the book has all come about through extensive research, personal experience and observation throughout many years. I have compiled this to make it simpler to understand the principles of nutrition and health. I hope this will enlighten you; and help you gain (better) insight into your own health, and that of your family.

You are being affected by the foods you are eating, and, the foods you are not eating!

Most illnesses have signs of nutrition and enzyme deficiency. Even the humble arthritis has a base of deficiency inherent and of excess of the wrong foods as the root of the cause.

As we are human we also have human traits to enjoy all aspects of life and not always be so regiment in our approaches to life. One golden rule stands out for me – 70/30 rule. Basically, one needs to consume wholesome foods 70% of the time the other 30% you can indulge in some way, with the objective to maintain this balance as much as possible .
Strive to achieve better health of the body, (and mind), and you will make a huge difference in life for the most important person, you, and for those around you!

It is a well known fact among the doctors and other medical personnel that it is easier to spend ten minutes administering chemotherapy on a cancer patient, (that costs $1,000 plus), than it is to spend one hour discussing health issues and lifestyle factors with the patient and charging $200. (Hopefully before the illness has taken a strong hold on them). Chemotherapy does not cure cancer, it holts its progress – nature's foods heal and have for centuries!

Picture this scenario if you may:

Two people are off to hospital, both require lung transplants. One person was a heavy smoker, the other lived a near healthy life and did not smoke. Let's just say there is only one set of lungs available on the donor register. Now, if they both meet at the entrance doors to the hospital, which patient should go first – and why?

"There are tribal groups, and many others, throughout the world that do not get our modern day illnesses!" (I will mention this again in the book). I know of a family member when queried about their vegetable intake they emphatically stated that they have vegetables every week. When scrutinized more closely, this person has roast vegetables with a roast on Sundays. Now, I am not against this pattern of eating, however, this is not enough to keep the body operating at peak efficiency, let alone build a strong immune system that can stave off the toughest of diseases. (Remember my 70/30 rule)?

A good part of the overall aim of this book:
To bring awareness to the fact that we;
- consume insufficient correct foods
- consume excessive amounts of the wrong foods
- can improve our relationships with others

ADDENDUM

BODY PH LEVELS AND EXCESS ACIDITY ENVIRONMENTS.
Your body has a natural acid and alkaline balance which is measured by the 'pH' scale which everyone should have some understanding of. For the body to remain alive and healthy the blood needs to be slightly ALKALINE with a pH reading of 7.365

Your body always tries to maintain a balance, known as homeostasis, to aim for the correct pH level. Most foods we consume these days are acid forming in the body. Now, if your blood is even marginally acidic then, some interesting things take place;

1. The body will try to store acid waste in fat cells.
2. The body will draw on Calcium (an alkaline mineral in abundance, especially in the bones) and this depletion of Calcium can be seen as 'Arthritis' and similar modern day health problems.
3. This paves the way for modern day health problems to take hold.

Most modern-day ill health patterns are seen in an acidic body – they thrive in these conditions!

What is the theme of this brief discussion? To bring awareness to the fact that the foods we eat are contributing to our ill health, especially our modern-day illnesses.

Tip – Have your doctor request a blood test to check on pH levels so you can be aware of potential future health problems taking hold.

See also, 'Low Acid Diet Plan' for further points of view on this acid / alkaline balance.

Further tests of your blood can be performed to check for;

- Homocysteine (level of inflammation in your body, hence, contributing factor for blood pH levels to change)
- C-Reactive Protein – an indication of blood clotting factors, that are also seen alongside ill-health patterns.
- Fibrinogen – a protein used in the blood clotting process, platelet aggregation, hence blood thickening.

These will be mentioned again.

AN IMPORTANT NOTE ON BLOOD CLOTTING;

Red blood platelets have a normal negative and positive balance within the cell, like all other cells. Now, if the platelets are out of balance with their electrons, possibly due to free radical interference, thus an 'ATTRACTING' of other out of balance charged platelets, creating a clumping together of red blood cells, clotting to be exact, which can be seen as a sign of future health problems.

The 'result' of this clumping together is to place the presenting patient on blood thinners. This will help the problem – yet *we need to consider the cause of this clumping of red blood cells.*
Hint: Take Epsom Salts \(Magnesium Sulphate) and Bi-Carb of Soda (Sodium Carbonate) to help take out Chlorine and Phosphorus.

This area needs further medical research a I strongly believe what has been mentioned above; blood pH, blood acidity levels and blood clotting via negative charged cells, have much correlation to our modern day health problems and have been overlooked as the core of the problem. Can't see the forest for the trees' We need to consider the basics and look at toxins in our foods and pathogens taking hold – this includes the bad bacteria in our digestive system.

Section I
Concise Health Reference

(for common ailments and low acid diet plan)

A to Z Health Reference

How to use this section:

Use the A to Z alphabetical format to find your health ailment. I have included many interesting facts that may help you further in understanding ourselves and, I hope this helps you on your quest for better understanding and 'Health 4 Ever!

> **Please note: The information is for educational purposes only, you must not alter your lifestyle, medication, exercise schedule, etc before seeking advice from your health professional. It is not intended to provide self-diagnosis, treatment or cure for any diseases. The writer, or any affiliates, accepts neither liability nor responsibility to any person or entity as a result of using information provided herein.**

Living a healthier life is not rocket science and does not require drastic changes to your lifestyle – just a few adjustments can make all the difference. However, you must consume good quality foods ***most*** of the time for your body to operate correctly – the more consumption of natural foods the healthier you can be.

You can enjoy that piece of cake, or take away food, but your aim is to consume good nutritional food at least 70% of the time.

Addressing the cause and not the symptoms is the best outcome for resolving health problems. If the cause is not corrected you are wasting your money, time and, probably injuring the body further. Ensure your health professional addresses the cause and NOT the symptom!

A huge swing in attitudes of the way we address our health issues is being experienced to the acceptance that lifestyle can influence modern day diseases, including cancer, arthritis and many others.

(Hint – if you want to improve or maintain your health then eat foods that contain life energy!)

Acid / Alkaline balance (See also, 'Low acid diet plan.').

You need to maintain the correct balance between acid and alkaline conditions in the body. Consuming excess acid producing foods will inevitably cause the blood and body system to become over acidic. *This is where the conditions are ripe for major health problems to manifest.* The main foods causing this condition are; fast foods, fats, dairy products, red meats and foods prepared with additives. We are constantly bombarded by the media and food companies that their food is good for you or low in fat. This is not altogether correct. For recommended replacement foods see section, 'Low acid diet plan.'

Some further acid producing foods; meat, chicken, dairy products, margarine, salt, cashew, peanuts, and excess wheat to name a few. There is a difference between acidic foods and acid-forming foods. While some foods may taste acidic, they can have an alkalizing effect on the body. What determines the pH nature of food in the body is the metabolic end products when it is digested and the minerals absorbed into the bloodstream.

When your body is over acidic then what tends to happen is Calcium is leeched from the bones to help alkalize the body. In doing so we lose valuable Calcium from the bones and muscles. This can result in arthritic conditions (and many other health problems), taking hold.

Remedy to remove acid waste

Remove acid producing foods altogether and replace with alkaline foods - potatoes, apples, vegetables, onions, garlic, celery, cabbage, soy, almonds (excellent), and other nuts and grains in general, bananas, yoghurt, cranberry juice, lecithin and wheat grass juice. Apple cider vinegar (excellent), lemon juice and parsley is also effective so too is watermelon.

Find what good and healthy foods are available for your area and consume those daily and as *raw as possible*, as all forms of cooked foods are deficient of enzymes. Enzymes are essential for the body to function correctly and efficiently. They are found in natural, whole foods and not in most processed foods, fast foods and others

Ageing

(Hint: You are probably being affected by insufficient nutrition that contributes to ageing of cells of the body even though we may think we are eating well.)

The two main causes are;

1. **Free Radical assault.** Free radicals bind themselves to cells and cause cellular damage. This, in turn, also aids the development of degenerative diseases which age the body.
2. **Decline in anti-ageing hormones.** Hormones are biochemicals that are secreted by endocrine glands such as pituitary, thyroid, adrenals, pancreas, etc. Hormones are like messengers that influence the function of the cells and the body. These hormones can be influenced by nutrition, (and enzymes), from foods we consume and toxins.

These are linked to nutritional deficiency

Anti-ageing hormones HGH (Human Growth Hormone) – The 'fountain of youth" hormone that can be affected by many aspects of ill-health and the consequences are ageing bodies.

Signs of ageing

- **The brain:** Forgetfulness, short-term memory loss, slow thinking.
- **The Heart:** Shortness of breath on exertion, ankle swelling, low cardiac efficiency.
- **The Liver:** Less detoxification ability, lethargy, low immune system.
- **The Pancreas:** Less digestive enzymes, excessive insulin or inactive pancreas.
- **The Gastrointestinal tract:** indigestion, bloating, burping, more wind, and large abdomen.

- **The Adrenal glands:** less hormone production including dehydroepiandrosterone or DHEA.
- **The Reproductive system:** less sex hormones.
- **The bone:** Osteoporosis or fragile bone, bone ache, more frequent fractures.
- **The Muscle:** flabby and weak muscles.
- **The Skin:** Loss of elasticity, more wrinkles, thin skin, becoming rough and lack of shine.

Remedy

Ensure plenty of natural foods and less processed foods. Apply the 70/30 rule of lifestyle, (as I call it). That being consume natural foods 70% of the time and consume <u>the not-so-healthy</u> foods 30% of the time to reduce early ageing of the body.

Alkaline Environment

An alkaline environment is desirable for hormones to be accepted by the cells of the body. The pH of the human body is alkaline at about 7.34. It is this pH that our bodies **function properly.** When the body is acidic it tends to push this acidity out to the joints. A further point; cancer cells do not survive in an alkaline environment.

Attention Deficit Disorder (ADD)

(Hint – Lacking attention, (love), from one or both parents.)

Diet related trigger factors also, and these are related to processed foods and foods that contain additives – especially artificially coloured foods like soft drinks, candies and other food stuffs containing the above. If you love your children then do not let them indulge in these artificial foods! These foods are poisonous to our bodies! Cravings for sweet foods is usually a sign of a deficiency in a particular mineral or nutrient the body needs. (Do not confuse this with diabetes).

Remedy

Remove all forms of sugar from the diet. Pay close attention to diet, lifestyle and exercise. True parental love and attention will not go astray.

Allergies

(Hint - Allergies respond best once emotions are sorted out!)

Linked to congestion and toxin absorption of the large intestine. Digestion needs to be addressed as well. Digestive enzymes are essential before your food can be broken down so that the nutrients can enter the blood <u>without</u> causing allergies. Allergies can also result from cooked foods and the wrong foods - they destroy the enzymes in our digestive system.

Remedy

Improve the diet, clean the bowels and strengthen the immune system. Take Vitamin B, especially B12, and horseradish. Look at your emotions - find what it is that puts you off-balance and resolve it! An allergy test may be necessary to determine allergen affecting you. Fresh fruit and vegetables and plenty of PURE water are a requirement to have an effect on allergies. But, once again, you need to consider all the above points of therapy as well.

Food Allergies

Poor protein absorption can lead to food allergies – <u>have digestion checked by your health professional,</u> as low stomach secretions can adversely affect the assimilation of proteins, among other nutrients. Also, <u>consuming incorrect foods</u> has an effect. (See section on dairy allergies)

Hay fever

This is an allergic condition of the mucous membranes of the eyes, ears and nose and linked with the immune system. Your diet needs improving. I have seen major improvements in symptoms – yes, you can eliminate hay fever!

Remedy

REMOVE dairy products totally! Take raw garlic, parsley and fenugreek. Ensure bowels are moving freely. A cleanse may be needed to move out old waste that may have accumulated. Minerals such as; Magnesium Phosphate, Sodium Chloride and Silica can address hay fever as well, your health shop can help here.

Note: If supplementing with vitamin tablets ensure you source quality products from a reputable health shop not just a supermarket shelf.

Quick remedy for hay fever bout;

Large dose of Vitamin C powder (a teaspoon size contains 3 to 4 grams). This will offer short term assistance to quell the symptoms and sneezing. Lemon juice and water and melon juice will help to eliminate allergies. Your diet needs improving – see a reputable Naturopath or similar.

Alcohol

Consuming alcohol during or just after a meal interrupts the digestion process – it ferments the food. That is why the next day you may feel uncomfortable in the stomach, experience altered bowel movements, etc. If you have to then the best time to drink is on an empty stomach, before the meal. Have alcohol free days if you want to have a drink – avoid binge drinking! Alcohol increases inflammation in the body and upsets your normal sleep patterns at night. I have spoken with many who have experienced this when having a drink. This inflammation is seen as; puffy eyes, mucous congestion of the throat and nasal passages and others.

Alzheimer's Disease

Studies conducted in Germany indicated that increased oxidation is a feature of Alzheimer's disease and that low concentrations of the antioxidant vitamins E and C, are found in cerebrospinal fluid.

Remedy

Take folic acid and remove all aluminium containing products from your life! Replace your aluminium pots, use alternative toothpaste, use non aluminium based deodorants. Take anti-oxidants like Vitamin C powder, tomatoes, Selenium supplements, Vitamin E foods. Lemons are <u>excellent</u> for a digestive stimulant. Often seen with a Zinc deficiency. Consume more nuts, unsalted, especially Almonds, Hazel nut and Pistachios. Walnuts are similar in shape as our brains, and do support the function. (This is known as 'nature's signature). Note: Consult with your doctor if on blood thinning medication if taking vitamin E.

Antacids

Antacid preparations reduce acidity and increase the risk of pathogens colonizing. *<u>You need a strong acid barrier in your digestive system!</u>* Antacids are no good for your digestive system; address your diet, and chew celery during an acid reflux attack. Then you must address your nutrition and digestion. If your stomach and digestive system is not sufficiently acidic then you will not correctly digest nor assimilate foods correctly – resulting in health problems and allergies to name a few.

Antibiotics

Antibiotics kill viruses and bacteria and are mostly <u>indiscriminant on our body's natural, good bacteria</u>. Therefore, this affects our immune system compromising its efficiency. Long-term use of antibiotics is definitely not recommended.

Antioxidants

Plant based antioxidants greatly protect against chronic, degenerative diseases. Antioxidants, especially Vitamin C, mop up free radicals. Make sure you include a daily intake of natural Vitamin C and/or Calcium Ascorbate in powder form, along with the myriad of antioxidants found in <u>natural and ALL coloured fruits and vegetables</u>, nuts and grains. Other powerful antioxidants include Vitamins A, C, E, and minerals Zinc, Selenium and Glutathione.

Arthritis

<u>Cause</u> - generally caused by excessive consumption of extremely unbalanced foods, (excessively acid producing by-products), excessive red meats, sugar and dairy products and other processed foods, over a long period of time. These processed foods the body cannot deal with correctly and ends up irritating the internal balance giving further inflammation, etc. This results in a chronic acid condition of the blood. (see acid / alkaline section.) This tends to settle in the joints of the body. Arthritis is usually seen as inflammation of the body, excess toxins in the system and <u>a lack of some key nutrients</u>, especially essential fatty acids. You are consuming foods that are contributing to your health problem.

Remedy

- Step 1 - Clean up your diet and get rid of; fast foods, dairy products, and purine producing foods such as; heavy red meat, sardines, lamb's fry, etc. Eliminate constipation (see Bowels section).

Fresh fruit and vegetables, nuts and grains will clean out your system.
Remove processed foods. This includes packaged cereals, white bread, pastries, etc.
Calcium, Magnesium, Iron, Sodium (not salt), Potassium and Sulphates to clean excess Phosphorus (from chemicals inour foods). Sulphur containing foods also include; Onions, Broccoli, cabbage, etc. raw as possible! as excess wastes *are seen in arthritis sufferers.* Address

your diet, see acid / alkaline foods section and rid yourself of the pain of arthritis.

- Step 2 - Phytoestrogen foods like; Soy, celery, parsley, nuts (watch peanuts), whole grains, apples, cabbage (raw), leafy green vegetables (raw).
- Step 3 - Glucosamine Sulphate (500mg, 3 times a day). Vitamin C (in powder form), and Vitamin E, and drink sage tea daily instead of coffee or tea.
- Step 4 – Exercise!

Eliminate

Milk, sugar, cheese, margarine and red meats. Also, most vegetable oils are hydrogenated in the processing and solidify when cold – these are not good for us!

Use these oils instead

Linseed oil (must be fresh as possible), Extra virgin olive oil, grape seed oil.

Some oils are heavily processed so aim for the natural oils which you can source from your local farmer's market in your area.

Rheumatoid Arthritis

Commonly low in key nutrients. Seen as an inflammatory condition within the body. You need to detoxify your body to clean out the system, check your digestive process with your local Naturopath or nutritionist. Rheumatoid arthritis and little or no gastric acid (hypochlorhydria), go hand in hand. Also, check bacterial overgrowth in gut – this can be done with a pH test through your health practitioner. Check long term digestion / absorption problems and incorrect foods. Need Vitamin E, beta-carotene and Selenium (has anti-inflammatory properties). Grape seed extract – contains rich source of proanthocyanidins, a flavonoid compound, with strong antioxidant and collagen strengthening abilities.

FOODS - Alkaline fruits and vegs, to remove acid build up in joints. Eg; Celery, onions which help increase good fats in blood also.

Carrot and Beetroot grated is excellent to help support the body but, must avoid foods that contribute to arthritis.

OTHER – nuts and seeds for EFA content to reduce inflammation. (sunflower seeds, almonds, walnuts, pumpkin seeds) Eat 2 apples a day if you suffer from arthritis, rheumatism, gout.

Silica can treat arthritic type disease and can reverse degenerative bone diseases and is found in whole grains, Tahini, almonds and other seed foods, cucumbers, turnips, dates. *60-80% of arthritis sufferers would benefit from dietary manipulation.* Fish oils for anti-inflammatory diseases, especially arthritis, R.A. and gout. *(Must eliminate meat from diet to have a substantial effect.)*

Meat contains the type of fat that stimulates the production of inflammatory agents in the body.

4 food ways to beat R.A.
1. Look for allergic trigger foods –wheat, corn, dairy, meat.
2. Forgo meat, especially pork, beef, processed and smoked meats, salami, etc.
3. Eat oils fish – contain anti-inflammatory agents, and include some ginger and turmeric as regular as possible.
4. Cut back on Omega 6 oils – margarines, safflower, sunflower, canola, corn. These are generally, hydrogenated oils, are also acid producing – something you don't want.

Remedy for aches and pains

Rub Wintergreen oil into affected area. The oil penetrates deep and is of great assistance in reducing inflammation. This oil also contains salicylates, which are natural painkillers similar to aspirin, only natural. Avoid NSAIDS (anti-inflammatory drugs), as these interfere with the digestive system contributing to gastrointestinal upset, and can be linked to some headaches and ulcers. Dry eyes can be a sign of arthritis.
Osteoporosis

Osteoarthritis (OA) degenerative joint disease indicated in age, injury, genetics and wear and tear. Morning joint stiffness is often the first symptom.

Remedy

- Limit animal proteins (or eliminate for a period),
- Eliminate sugar and refined carbohydrates

Reason

These substances mentioned, chelate (remove) calcium out of the body. Calcium is an alkaline mineral and where excess acidity is seen in the body, then calcium is 'used' to help neutralize. In turn, the bones lose calcium – the joints gain acid waste. (This is a very simple explanation to the process of Osteoporosis.)

Excess acidity seen in the body.
  Increase
- Vegs. (but watch nightshades – potatoes, eggplant, tomatoes, capsicum initially). Consume Omega 3 oils in fish, linseeds. Consume more berries, cherries, pineapple, bananas. Avoid processed foods. Weight gain puts further stress on joints. Zinc and Vitamin C are needed for the synthesis and stability of collagen. (Collagen is the core and base of bone structure).

Summary of Prevention factors:

- Limit phosphate rich foods – processed meats, cheeses, soft drinks.
- Eat lots of vegetables
- Include sufficient fibre (wholegrain cereals and pasta)
- Include yoghurt daily – a tablespoon a day is good
- Drink sufficient water daily to help hydrate and flush the cells of the body
- AVOID Aluminium products and cooking utensils, especially deodorants

- Limit meat intake – stir fry dishes are good they use less meat
- Limit sugar and salt (eliminate them), limit instant coffee intake – try some nutritious herbal teas.
- **No white bread!**
- Eliminate foods that contribute ; these include processed, fatty, salty foods, (the body cannot process these correctly.)

Herbal – Ginger, anti-inflammation, Garlic, Turmeric.

TURMERIC – 1200mg of curcumin has the same anti-arthritis activity as 300mg of the anti-inflammatory drug phenylbutazone.

Rheumatoid Arthritis and little or no gastric acid (hypochlorhydria), go hand in hand. Check bacterial growth in gut.(See your health professional). Chili (Capsaicin) relieves arthritis and can, along with other foods, address cancer.

Asthma

(NOTE: Please see your Health Practitioner as asthma can be life threatening.)

A vegan diet to cleanse and strengthen the system is paramount – this should be done for several weeks at least. Address the diet, especially processed foods and additives; check digestion as most asthmatics have compromised digestive capabilities. Remove margarine and meat, the alternatives are Tahini and lentils, almonds and other nuts, as these foods are not acid producing for the body. Drink lots of PURE clean water daily!

Childhood asthma - Most asthmatic children have poor digestion and poor diet patterns.

- Address diet, especially processed foods and additives.
- Drink lots of PURE clean water daily!

Then take; Vitamin C 1000mg, 3 times a day, 1 tablespoon of cod liver oil, 1 high potency Vit. / Min. capsule 3 times a day.

Addressing the diet means consuming fresh, natural vegetables and fruit, daily avoiding the obvious. See, 'Low acid diet plan' for more information.

Diet aside, what type of asthma do you have; mechanical, or physiological. Anxiety, concern and panic all produce muscular contractions. Most asthmatics have poor digestive secretions of the stomach which should be addressed with a consultation with your local Naturopath or similar.

Back

(Hint - the more physically active you are the better shape your back, and body, will be in. See section on basic back care for more information).
Most back complaints tend to be <u>muscle spasms</u> rather than actual physical damage to the back structure. You will have to check with a qualified health professional.

We find that 80% of injuries occur because of inflexibility of the body [and mind]. Exercise regularly. When back pain strikes we tend to shy away from exercise when the very thing is to keep mobile. Try Yoga, Tai Chi or some form of stretching and strengthening therapy.

> Many back complaints are centered on muscle spasms more so than actual physical injury to the back. To give an example of a muscle spasm; walking down steps you miss the step and stumble to the next step and you feel your back twinge a little. The strong tendons have tried to save your back and tightened up considerably, likened to a twisted rope, and have placed pressure on other structures of the back. This is not always the case yet I have experienced this many times myself. A masseur or professional trained in care of the back can help.

The key to improving back complaints;
Loosen mobility muscles, tighten stability muscles, loosen tight nerves and mobilise stiff joints. Please read this again and think about

what you are reading and what it means to you. Visit your local gym, Pilates class, etc. for help.

Stability muscles stabilise the joint, for example; while we are sitting, and mobility muscles move the joint through its range, for example; when playing sports.

Strengthen deep stability muscles by;
1. Exercising at low levels
2. Use <u>prolonged holds</u> to engage stability muscles.

After injury stability muscles remain weak until you retrain them. Posture is very often overlooked when it comes to back problems: Remain conscious of your posture STAND TALL! (See section on back care.)

Blood

(Hint: The plant kingdom is good for our health. A molecule of blood and a molecule of plant chlorophyl has the same structure except in the centre - blood has a molecule of iron and chlorophyl has a molecule of Magnesium.)

Beetroot is nature's excellent blood purifier. A TRULY wonderful healer for many modern day illnesses and complaints. Contains high contents of; Iron, Copper, Manganese, Vitamin C – <u>all blood builders.</u>

Hawthorn berries reduce stickiness of blood, as does olive oil. Olive oil contains more oleic acid (the dominant fatty acid in olive oil), and less arachidonic fatty acid that encourages stickiness. Olive oil benefits platelet function

Thin blood carries nutrients and oxygen more efficiently to all the cells of the body.

Thick blood cannot carry nutrients to all the cells of the body. Remember that cancer thrives in an anaerobic environment.

Blood Platelet Aggregation (Blood Clotting)

Garlic and the onion family, fish oils, Vitamin E and Ginkgo Biloba lower blood viscosity and inhibit platelet aggregation. Green Tea is also good. So is Olive oil, Chinese black mushrooms, and Ginger. Linseed oil cold pressed is also good. Other blood thinning foods – the onion family, Chinese black mushroom. (known as; mo-er or 'tree ear') is known as a longevity tonic.

<u>Fibrinogen (a protein used in blood clotting process), if excess in blood then can be lowered by;</u> 2,000 mg a day of Vitamin C, 1,000mg of flush-free Niacin, 2,800mg of EPA/DHA from fish oil, and 2,000mg a day of bromelain. Some practitioners suggest low-dose Aspirin, Vitamin E, and garlic, along with Ginkgo Biloba and green tea extracts to protect against a fibrinogen induced arterial blood clot, of which could cause a stroke.

Blood Vessels

High concentrations of bioflavonoids (esp fruit), strengthen blood vessel walls and help prevent them rupturing. Vitamin C is involved in the synthesis of glycosaminoglycans, chemicals that inhibit blood clotting and <u>are components of the linings of blood vessels.</u>

Blood sugar levels unstable

Regular meals of complex carbohydrates and protein will help to rebalance as will regular exercise. Ensure good levels of amino acids are in your diet, Spirulina is good.

Blood Viscosity

Tobacco smoking raises blood viscosity and increase the chance of blood-clot formation.
Trans fatty acids, especially processed foods with these fats in them, thicken the blood also. These are not the only contributors just pay attention to the 'foods' you put in your mouth.

Strokes

Reduce the chance of strokes and lower blood viscosity levels it is important to maintain adequate intake of Vitamins C and E, Selenium, Magnesium, Calcium, Potassium, and

Blood thinning foods

Onions, Vitamin C, garlic, fish oil and Bioflavonoids.
Magnesium foods – Oatmeal, whole meal bread, peas, yoghurt, avocadoes, bananas, oranges, figs, peaches. Potassium foods – Oatmeal, yoghurt, tomatoes, prunes, figs, avocadoes, broccoli, carrots, oranges, bananas, peaches. Two bananas a day – 66mg Magnesium and 23mg Potassium. 1 tub of yoghurt a day for Calcium is helpful.

Atheroma (Coronary Artery Lesions)

If the bloodstream has a high concentration of antioxidants, especially Vitamins C and E, it is more difficult for the oxidation reaction to occur. Any internal inflammation process has to be further investigated by your health professional.

Blood Cholesterol

Should be within the range of 4.0mmol/L and not allowed to rise above 6.0mmol/L.

Blood clots

Bromelain in pineapples helps dissolve blood clots. Garlic and onions in general, are beneficial. Vitamin C and fish oil, and include Linseed oil.

Blood tests – things to check (ask your doctor to check these and explain what they indicate).

Levels of

- Homocysteine,
- Cholesterol (both LDL and HDL)

- <u>DHEA, C-Reactive protein</u> (stroke indicator and heart attack),
- <u>Fibrinogen</u> and plasma carotenoid. Request these on your next visit to your doctor – please!
- <u>pH level of your blood</u>

Blood Pressure (see High Blood Pressure)

(Please note; blood pressure signs can be hard to gauge so please consult your physician.)

Some signs can be; morning headache, nosebleeds, dizziness, ringing in the ears, fainting spells, blurred vision, depression, urinating at night.

Important to keep BP below 140/90, especially for the older person. One side effect of high BP is strokes. See high blood pressure.

Body Odour

Usually caused by the incorrect foods being consumed in combination with poor elimination. Often seen when there is a lack of Silica in the diet. More natural foods like fruits and vegetables needed and less heavy, processed foods. The elimination channels of the body, skin, bowels, lungs, etc are not functioning normally.

Bowels

Natural laxative foods – Figs, dates, grapes, raisins, currants, plums and prunes. Other 'black' type foods are good for bowel.

Doctrine of signatures – black (liquorice, prunes, plums, etc.) to remove 'black' waste from the body. Like cures like signature in foods.

Herbs – liquorice, cascara, aloes, senna, molasses. Senna Pod infusion is good to cleanse the bowel. Celery, Silver beet, beetroot are good vegetables to scour bowel pockets and flexures. Linseed and Olive oil are good to assist the sliding action of bowel contents.

Colon cancer usually seen in three areas; cecum, sigmoid colon and rectum. Keep them clean and for further advice speak to your Natural Therapist.

A short fast (1 full day at least) is good for the digestive system. Slippery elm is good, you cannot overdo this herb.

Fibre – the importance of

Fibre in the colon binds and dilutes bile acids, which have been implicated in the promotion stage of colon cancer.

Dietary fibre, in addition to binding to bile salts and producing cancer-fighting butyric acid, another component of fibre, phytic acid also protects against cancer of the colon. Phytic acid found in fibre, is a natural plant antioxidant in most cereals, legumes and nuts. Usually 1 – 5% is found, but is not in fruit, potatoes and starch foods.

Epidemiological international surveys indicate that the rate of <u>colon cancer decreases when the diet is rich in phytic acid.</u>

Absorption

Packaging of foods, for example breakfast cereals, may list a certain iron content per serving but do not provide enough information as to bioavailability. Bioavailability is the ability of our digestive systems to absorb and utilise the nutrient, and everyone can be different, especially as we age. So, if the packaging says, "10mg of zinc" we may only be absorbing a fraction of this.

Indigestion

Try a little Ginger in hot water and sip. Address the foods you consume.

Remedy

Raw fruits and vegetables and reduce heavy processed foods and this will help.

Senna Pod infusion is good to cleanse the bowel. Celery, Silver beet, beetroot are good vegetables to scour bowel pockets and flexures. Linseed and Olive oil are good to assist the sliding action of bowel contents.

Colon cancer usually seen in three areas; cecum, sigmoid colon and rectum. Keep them clean and for further advice speak to your Natural Therapist, or health practitioner.

Natural remedies;

Aloe Vera juice – stomach ulcers, colitis, Irritable Bowel syndrome

Psyllium Husks – bowel cleansing, removes stagnant waste, short term recommended. Digestive herbs – parsley, ginger, aniseed, dill. Digestion and flatulence – cumin, tumeric, ginger, coriander, caraway.

Irritable Bowel Syndrome – Olive leaf extract is effective.

Bad breath linked to constipation. Can also be intestinal parasites, (Helicobacter Pylori)

This parasite is more common than you think and attaches itself to the lining of the stomach causing irritation. Chickpeas, coriander and pumpkin seed kernels help to rid the body of this aggressive parasite.

A short fast (1 full day at least) is good for the digestive system. Slippery elm is good, you cannot overdo this herb.

Intestinal Transit Time (ITT) is the time it takes for ingested food to pass through the intestinal tract and out. This should be **up to eighteen hours and no more than twenty-four hours.** What this means is that the bowel movement you have today, should be from food you ate yesterday.

- If your bowels are slow then the body is absorbing toxins. You will see health conditions improve when your bowels are moving correctly. This is so important to keep you in better health.

How to check your ITT

With your next meal eat some corn but don't chew some of the corn kernels. Most digestive systems cannot digest the outer layer of the corn, so some of them will pass through undigested. You will see them in your stools and this will give you an indication how quick, or slow, your bowels take to clear. If your bowels are too quick you may not be digesting foods correctly and receiving the nutritional benefits: If your bowels are slow then you will be absorbing toxins and waste that should be discarded quickly to avoid re-absorption.

Remedy

For sluggish bowels try iron foods plus sprouts, brown rice, vegetables, fruits, etc.

The best remedy for constipation is fruits and vegetables, especially fruits like pears and apples among the many that have great benefits to cleanse the intestines and the body as a whole. Raw is best!

Try these also; dates, prunes, etc.

Most all bowel problems can be improved by paying attention to the following;

- Consume foods that are raw, whole and unprocessed
- Eliminate coffee, alcohol, sugar, and red meats especially and processed saturated fatty foods.
- Regular exercise
- Relaxation methods including meditation, Yoga, Tai Chi, etcetera.

Use other methods also mentioned in this section on bowels to address problems.

BOWEL CLEANSE required as this area can be a major problem. Take; Omega3 fatty acids, Vitamin C, B6, A and D. Ideally a vegan diet and improving digestion are paramount. Herbs to use; Sage, Gentian, Mullein, Thyme, Licorice, Fenugreek and Horseradish.

Biochemical remedy- Potassium Phosphate, Magnesium Phosphate (nerve nutrients), and Potassium Chloride (Blood conditioner.)

Cancer

CAUTION:(Please see your qualified health practitioner for advice on cancer treatment.)

Hint – Most people think that cancer is related to your genes when, in fact, most cancers are related to your lifestyle.

An interesting comment:

"Caused by excessive accumulation of toxins in the body, <u>and seen as a nutrient deficiency problem</u>".

Chemical exposure (and toxicity) can compromise the immune system, allowing pathogens to take hold, thus, allowing **altered DNA replication** to take over a once normal system.

Cancer seems to be an altered or damaged DNA 'based' illness and resulting in abnormal growth patterns.

Cancer seen as chemical/ viral driven, then DNA damage leading to mutation of genes & deformed / altered genes.

What else can you do? The following is essential;

- Eliminate beef and pork, eliminate meats and replace with seeds and nuts   (see note below)
- Removal of solid (saturated) oils, including margarine and other hydrogenated oils
- Drink more pure water!
- Consume more fibre
- Avoid processed foods
- Consume foods high in phytochemicals; blue, black, raspberries and strawberries and pomegranates*
- Avoid processed foods (yes, I have mentioned it again)
- Reduce soft drinks and cordials, (artificial colours and other chemicals)
- Eliminate processed and de-natured foods

Note to 'Eliminate meats' – Excess animal protein depletes the Pancreas of KEY enzymes that are seen to address cancer cells in the body. Excess animal protein is acidic for the body and slows the bowels – two things that cancer cells like!

Research shows that most cancers can be addressed somewhat with dietary manipulation!

What to do first

Complete and correct cleansing and detoxing of the body!
Anticancer foods

Raspberries, Pomegranates, Turmeric, Tomatoes, Broccoli (esp Sprouts), Cabbage. Peas, beans, soya bean, lentils.

Apple seeds and Apricot kernels, have strong anti-cancer capabilities.

OTHERS;

- Address sodium / potassium balance – this is done with foods, especially fruit and vegs, and eliminate salt.
- Oxygen rich blood (thin blood), as more oxygen in blood less likelihood of cancer developing. Cancer will not survive in an oxygen rich environment.
- Acid / Alkaline balance – Cancer thrives in an acid environment. Addressed with natural fruit and vegs. Some more specific than others. Eg; Water Melon.
- Eliminate saturated fats replace with Omega3's from fish and EFA's from Linseed oil, nuts, grains, no margarine!

Foods that fight Cancer

Allium containing foods;
- Garlic, onions, leeks, chives, shallots
- Cruciferous containing foods;
- **Broccoli,** cauli, cabbage, brussels sprouts, asian greens (eg. Bok Choy)
- Green Leafy vegetables;
- Spinach, silverbeet, dark green and purple lettuce
- Red/Orange coloured;
- **Beetroot,** carrots, sweet potatoes, pumpkin, red capsicum, tomatoes, rock melon, peaches, apricots, mangoes
- Berries;
- Strawberries, raspberries, blackberries, blueberries
- Citrus;
- Oranges, lemons, limes, grapefruit, mandarins,

Broccoli, beetroot (raw), cauli, cabbage, Brussels sprouts, turnips, radishes, spring greens are excellent. Sulphur compounds like diallyl sulphide, isothiocyanates and dithiolthiones, which are present in cruciferous vegetables (<u>especially sulforaphane in broccoli</u>) and in <u>Allium plants</u> like onion and garlic are highly protective against cancer.

Umbelliferous vegetables (carrots, celery, parsnips) contain antioxidants and other chemicals that protect against cancer.

Raspberries and pomegranates contain ellagic acid, and these have an effect on cancer cells dividing.

Cabbage (esp green leaves) contain an angiostatin enzyme that helps stop blood vessels growing into the cancer. Suggestion is to include more of these foods in your daily nutrition plan.(Please read this statement again).

You can consume a good handful of raspberries and cabbage a day.

Garlic – lowers risk of cancers of stomach and digestive system. Indoles, in cruciferous vegetables, block estrogen receptor sights in breast cancer cells. Broccoli – most important indole is indole-3-carbinol.

Can you see how nature can offer assistance in the fight against cancer?

Vitamin B17 (Laetrile)

Apricot Kernel and bitter almonds have the highest concentration. B17 is strong cancer cell fighter. Other sources are; alfalfa, linseed, broad beans, lima beans, garlic, soya beans, BERRIES, black strap molasses, macadamia nuts, sprouts, rice, rye, oats, millet, **seeds of apples, plum, cherry, and apricots.**

EAT THE SEEDS OF THE COMMON FRUIT

- Cancer prevention and reversion – you need EFA's (strong antioxidants), mackerel, salmon, tuna, crustaceans, sardines no added oil.
- Extra antioxidant foods – strawberry, apple, tomato, red grape, orange(include pith), lemon, mandarin, onions including raw garlic.
- Detoxify free radicals – cruciferous veg; broccoli, cauli, Brussels sprouts, cabbage especially green leaves less cooked as possible.
- Nutritional supplementation – Vits A, C, E, beta carotene, selenium, folic acid, Co-Enzyme Q10, BIOFLAVONOIDS.

The real heroes in the war against cancer are FRUITS and VEGETABLES!

Lung Cancer – usually shows the strongest association with low levels of beta carotene. One does not need to mention stop smoking if you are a smoker.

Breast Cancer

Do not consume fats, especially animal fats, including cheese, butter and meat fat. Such fat may spur a recurrence of the cancer after it is surgically removed.

Dairy products may aggravate cysts and lumps of the breast. Dietary fat prodded the growth of new tumours that are oestrogen dependent. Studies now reveal this to be so.

Further; *the theory is that high fat diets boost blood concentrations of oestrogen that becomes fuel to feed the growth of further tumours.*

(Please read the previous statement again)

Diet prescription against breast cancer.

- Cruciferous vegetables are vital to assist in burning up excess oestrogen so less is available to feed cancer. Indole 3 Carbinol is a compound in cruciferous vegetables that helps deactivate this excess oestrogen that seems to be at the centre of breast cancer.
- Lots of vegetables and fruit (as raw as possible), Omega 3 fats from fish and Linseed oil.
- Eliminate margarine and use avocado for spreads.
- Eliminate dairy products and de-natured, processed foods

Soya bean products which contain plant oestrogens (phytoestrogens) that bind to oestrogen receptors on breast tissue can be effective.

Beans are excellent as they contain phytoestrogens that help block the activity of cancer-promoting oestrogen. **CoQ10 enzyme** shows good benefits in protection from breast cancer. It seems to be the case that breast cancer cases double in post menopausal women who consumed the least carotenoids. Carotenoids are found in leafy green vegetables, yellow vegetables like carrots and pumpkin to name a few.

Bowel Cancer

Foods that seem to promote bowel cancer include; excess meat consumption and alcohol consumption, low fibre foods and high fat diets. A balanced diet will see you consuming more fruits vegetables and nuts and less meat. *(Note: Meat does not contain much fibre and tends to stay in the digestive tract for a longer time. Toxins are further absorbed into the system.)*
Foods that help include; vegetables, especially cruciferous veg. like cabbage, broccoli, cauliflower. Seafood and foods high in fibre, Calcium and Vitamin D. Vitamin C and E can reduce faecal mutagens and help protect bowel linings.
People with low levels of Folic acid and high alcohol intake increase risk of colorectal cancer due to DNA damage. Learn to control your intake putting aside <u>days of alcohol free times</u> and eat correctly to strengthen the body.

Stomach Cancer

Nitrosamines are the specific cause of stomach cancer, and a major cause of cancer of the oesophagus. Pickled foods, preserved and cured meats, and dried salted fish all correlate with the incidence of stomach cancer.

The damage done to the epithelium and that eventually leads to stomach cancer 30 to 50 years later, usually happens in the first decade of life.

Foods good for stomach – red clover, carrot, cruciferous vegetables, (Red Clover is excellent due to their phyto-oestrogen content; genistein and daidzein.) Green Tea is claimed to protect against cancers of the skin, stomach and lung.

Prostate Cancer

High intake of vitamins C and K have a lower risk of men developing prostate cancer. This combination reduces cancer cell activity. Cancer cells prefer anaerobic environments. <u>Exercise will greatly assist reducing the impact of cancer cells</u> as we exercise we increase oxygen content in the blood – this is why exercise is SO important for your health. Lycopene found mainly in tomatoes is very helpful.

6 Quick Tips – Eating to avoid cancer.
1. Cut back on fats – remove trans fats (seen in take away foods, pastries + others
2. Eat more fruit and vegetables
3. Control your weight
4. Eat more fibre
5. Less salt, minimal consumption of cured and smoked foods and watch char-grilled foods
6. Drink alcohol in moderation and stop smoking immediately

Herbal – Basil, **Red Clover**, Lemongrass, rosemary, Tarragon, TURMERIC.
Bromelain, Curcumin, Cayenne Pepper, Liquorice (the Triterpenoids in liquorice may stifle quick growing cancer cells.

Plant based diets protect against cancer! Many health (cancer) research centres are finding this in studies conducted throughout the world.
Chromium and Vanadium almost always missing in cancer sufferers. Supplementation can have incredible reversing effects.

What else can you do?
The following is essential;
- Eliminate beef and pork, eliminate meats and replace with seeds and nuts
- Removal of solid (saturated) oils, <u>including margarine</u>
- Drink more pure water!

- Take charcoal to help rid body of toxins and waste
- Consume more fibre
- Avoid processed foods
- Consume foods high in phytochemicals
- Consume blue, black, raspberries and strawberries
- <u>Avoid processed foods</u> (yes, I have mentioned it again)
- Reduce soft drinks and cordials, (artificial colours and other chemicals)

If you are serious about your health then take control of your life now!

Weight & Cancer

Being overweight increases the risk of cancer, particularly cancers of the womb, oesophagus, kidney and gall bladder. Studies suggest that 15-20% of cancers are through being overweight alone.

Physical activity and Cancer

Being physically inactive has emerged as a big risk, especially of the breast and bowel cancer. Regular exercise is the key, and remember – to lose weight, increase the intensity and/or reduce the calories. Try walking twice a day. Organise your schedule to include an exercise regime. You don't want to suffer a major health problem unnecessarily, do you? Vary the intensity to assist in rebooting your metabolism level.

- Chemical Exposure, in its various forms, can alter DNA of the cells. Example; Weedkiller sprayed on to weeds, these die down then some shoot with altered growth structure – mutagenic process, the leaves are deformed. Many chemicals are usedto produce our 'foods'
- Compromised immune system – therefore allowing pathogens to take hold, hence; pathogenic driven sub-health problems.
- Nutrition requirements are heightened at this stage and possibly not addressed.

- Inflammation is often seen in excess, the body is fighting something, blood starts to clot, then we administer blood thinners. We need to address the cause and look further into the cause of this inflammation.
- Genetics – a weakness in the genes carried through to following generations, that we need to be aware of and take steps before cancertakes hold. If you have a family history of cancers,etc. then have your doctor request tests be done regularly before they take hold. Can you do something about genetic driven cancers?Yes, get tested regularly – this your doctor needs to take a little more care and request them.

Processed foods - the number one problem in western society is the consumption of processed foods that the body cannot deal with correctly. They may taste great and look good but think about what you are putting into your body.

Cancer is prevalent since introduction of artificial fertilisers, applied to soils, resulting in excess **Phosphorus** In our bodies, hence, toxicity and altered DNA. Eliminate foods grown with these chemicals and eat organic!

Some further theory

When a group of cancer cells detaches from the host tumour and enters the blood, most cells (99.9%) will be destroyed by the natural killer cells of the <u>immune surveillance system.</u>
If some escape, they immediately begin to excrete proteolytic enzymes, such as hyaluronidase, that digest and dissolve tissue so the cancer can continue to grow.
<u>*Platelet aggregation is necessary for metastised cells to adhere to the new host tissue*</u>, so blood factors that inhibit platelet aggregation are an important defense against the spread of cancer.

Foods that inhibit aggregation; Garlic, fish oils, Vitamin E and Ginkgo biloba lower blood viscosity and inhibit platelet aggregation. Avoid the foods that do the opposite, that is; thicken the blood, cause inflammation, etc.

Vitamin Therapy for cancer

Vitamin C is involved in the synthesis of glycosaminoglycans, chemicals that inhibit blood clotting and <u>are components of the linings of blood vessels.</u>

- **Vitamin C not only promotes collagen synthesis, making it more difficult for the tumour to invade surrounding tissue, but it <u>deactivates hyaluronidase</u>, one of the main enzymes excreted by a tumour to dissolve tissue.**

Vitamin C (and fibre) especially useful in the prevention of stomach cancer because it <u>blocks the transformation of amines and nitrites into nitrosamines</u>. Nitrosamines from pickled and preserved meats, for example; bacon, salami, hot dogs, are the most ubiquitous and potent dietary carcinogens.
Vitamin C helps to neutralise free radical cancer causing agents in cell membranes, addressing the first stage of cancer.

Selenium Taking 200mcg a day has been demonstrated to reduce the risk of prostate cancer by 74%, colon cancer by 60% and lung cancer by 30%. Selenium works with Vitamin E to help prevent cancer.
Folic acid. People with low levels of Folic acid and high alcohol intake increase risk of colorectal cancer due to DNA damage.

Foods that promote blood clotting;
SMOKING and fatty foods, especially those that contain trans fats that are found in pastries, thickeners, etc. Also, processing foods can add to the thickening of the blood.

Cancer and Free Radical Theory

Free radicals are unstable atoms capable of damaging DNA of the cell, the more free radical damage to DNA the more abnormal cells are created. Research has revealed that those who do not eat enough fruits and vegetables **regularly** are *twice as much in danger of developing cancer later in life.*

7 main indicators of symptoms
- Unusual bleeding or discharge
- Appearance of a lump or swelling
- Hoarseness or cough
- Indigestion or difficulty swallowing
- Change in bowel or bladder habits
- A sore that does not heal
- A change in a wart or mole

How to prevent cancer and treat it nutritionally
(This is for educational purposes only – you must see your doctor.)

Remove risk factors
Highly processed foods and foods devoid of much nutritional and enzymatic content, excessive alcohol consumption, high fat diet, high red meat intake, chemical laden foods, environmental factors (see notes at end), smoking, stress, and others.

Diet high in antioxidants
Fruits and vegetables, and their juices. Strawberries, apple, tomato, red grape, orange, lemon, mandarin, and onion are excellent sources of antioxidants.

Nutritional Supplementation
Ensuring the body receives correct amounts of vitamins, trace elements and antioxidants to prevent free radical damage. We must protect the DNA from oxidative damage by taking antioxidants.
Vitamins; **A**, (betacarotene) **C, E, Selenium, Folic acid, Co-EnzymeQ10, and bioflavonoids are all excellent.** Include N-Acetyl L-Cysteine and Glutathione.

Anti-cancer agents (that act as blockers and suppressors) are;
Class 1. Vitamin C; indoles and isothiocyanates from cruciferous vegetables; organosulphur compounds from garlic, onions, and other Allium vegetables; citrus fruit oils.
Class 2. Glutathione, organosulphur compounds from Allium vegetables; dithiolthiones from cruciferous vegetables.
Class 3. Vitamin E; isothiocyanates from cruciferous vegetables; dilemonene from orange oil.

Inflammation

Inflammation reactions are necessary for metastised cancer cells to attach themselves to host tissue.
Anti-inflammatory agents include; linseed and fish oils, garlic, ginger, cruciferous vegetables, etc. Many carcinogens cause damage by weakening the immune system, and it is extremely important to keep the immune system strong and efficient..
Cancer prevention; choose a plant-based diet that includes a rich variety of vegetables, fruits, nuts, pulses and minimally processed starchy foods. Use modest amounts of oils but concentrate on olive, walnut, grape seed, for the anti inflammation benefits also. People who ignore nutrition in helping their cancer, are limiting their ability to improve their health – nutrition is a good source of therapy for cancer.

40% of male cancers are dietary related and 60% of female cancers are diet related. Diet is therapeutic for cancer and is 'now' well supported that this will make a huge difference.
Plasma Carotenoid tests measures the amount of blood carotenoids in the system. This is a blood test performed by your doctor that measures the level of vegetables, to put it plainly, in your system. This has a correlation in cancer therapy the higher the level of vegetables in your diet (blood) the lesser prevalence of cancer cells to some degree.

Acid conditions can be the breeding ground for disease including tumours and cancers and other blood diseases – think about the consequences of what you eat **most of the time.**

Cancer – summarized

"Most people think that cancer is related to your genes when, in fact, cancer is related to your lifestyle!"

I have mentioned this again and for very good reason.

What to do first

<u>Complete and correct cleansing and detoxing of the body!</u>
Cancer cells prefer anaerobic environments. <u>Exercise will greatly assist reducing the impact of cancer cells</u> as we exercise we increase oxygen content in the blood – this is why exercise is SO important for your health.

Physical activity and Cancer

Being physically inactive has emerged as a big risk, especially relating to breast and bowel cancer. Regular exercise is the key, and lose weight, increase the intensity and/or reduce the calories. Try walking twice a day and include a brisk session where you stretch out your stride. Organise your schedule to include an exercise regime. You don't want to suffer a major health problem unnecessarily, do you? Vary the intensity to assist in rebooting your metabolism level.

4 areas to address to combat or eliminate cancer
1. Reduce the heavily processed foods (pastries, white bread, margarine, etc.) from your nutritional plan and increase raw fruits and vegetables
2. Take Pancreatic Enzymes (Pineapple has enzyme that mimics these enzymes)
3. Take Vitamin B17 (found in seeds of common fruits, esp. Apricot kernels, cherries, etc)
4. Toxins – remove **all** sources including <u>processed foods</u>, skin and hair care
5. Ensure adequate intake of KEY vitamins and minerals
6. Fresh fruits and vegetables in their natural state constantly!

Do see a reputable health practitioner that can guide you with correct lifestyle changes and correct foods to consume and those to avoid.

Add to this;
- Limit animal protein (this taxes the pancreas), ensure good digestion <u>and absorption</u> (see digestion section)
- B17 is also known as Laetrile, and is found in Apricot kernels, millet, cashews and spelt. B17 also needs an enzyme to activate the process and this is released by healthy pancreas, and, can be mimicked by bromelain in pineapples. Eat the seeds of the common fruit is mentioned in the bible, Genesis 1 /29. The seeds are loaded with all the right nutrients for our bodies (and live enzymes!)

Final Points on Cancer
- The induction time for most cancers is 15 to 30 years – cancer is really a disease of the young.
- Not consuming enough fruits and vegetables regularly can see the risk of developing cancer double later in life.

Cancer is prevalent since introduction of artificial fertilisers, applied to soils, resulting in excess **Phosphorus** In our bodies, hence, toxicity and altered DNA. Eliminate foods grown with these chemicals and eat organic!

Cataracts

A condition of the eye. Also seen as halo around lights. This is also a sign of liver disfunction.

Remedy

Vitamin C shows effective assistance and slows and reverses cataracts. Address what is causing this in the first place. This is not necessarily linked to 'OLD AGE'! Can be linked with free radical damage to the cells through incorrect nutritional factors. Consult your Naturopath or similar practitioner.

Celiac Disease

Is the reaction to gluten, the protein of wheat and rye, oats and barley. Causes tissue changes in the mucosal cells of the duodenum. Symptoms include; loss of weight, distension of the abdomen and steatorrhea, (fat in the stools).

Remedy – Remove gluten foods from the diet; <u>eat sufficient fresh fruit and vegetables</u>, dried fruit, nuts (no peanuts), and legumes.

Digestive Enzymes – pineapple, lettuce, chives, prunes

Foods to assist carbohydrate digestion – apples(pectin), pineapple, beans, cabbage, celery, parsley, carrots, spinach/silver beet, cucumbers, lettuce, garlic(raw), onions (lightly cooked raw if possible)
Brown Rice, polenta
Herbs – licorice, sage (esp. purple sage)
If low in iron then; pulvorise all green herbs in a blender, add lemon / pineapple juice (fresh), and enjoy the benefits.
Remove – fats, processed foods, margarine and dairy products, at least for the time being.

Chemicals to Avoid

Aspartame, Flouride, Mercury (also seen in tooth fillings)
Aluminium products to avoid also are; cooking pots, under arm deodorants containing aluminium. (These are not the only aluminium containing products though.)

Cholesterol

Found in animal foods, and is a big contributor to today's current health problems. Cholesterol is required for the brain function and, in fact, every cell of the body needs it. The problem with restricted blood flow in your arteries is not only excess 'bad' cholesterol, the problem also stems from oxidative stressors, such as free radicals and other factors that cause inflammation. The body will try to maintain clean arteries but if the immune system is not strong enough and you don't give the body as many tools for immune repair as for immune destruction, <u>the</u>

body will not have what it needs to fully repair damaged arterial walls. The lesions thus remain partially unhealed and plaque starts to build up in them. So, it seems, that this damage stems from inflammation, from free radical damage and leads to an accumulation of plaque.

Remedy

Can be controlled by the onion family – garlic, onions, chives, etc., raw and natural!
Raw Lecithin taken daily (available from health shops), garlic and onions as mentioned, taken regularly and in the natural form, will break down cholesterol. Beans, oat bran, oats (try them for breakfast), and pectin containing foods like apples. Oxidative damage and acid waste elements in the blood system irritate the delicate lining of the blood vessels causing damage that is 'patched up' by triglycerides & cholesterol. This thickens & narrows the arteries. Statins prescribed also reduce Co-enzyme Q10 which is critical for heart health!!

Margarine and other spreads

Margarine is acid forming for the body and is not really a food. Forget the hype of, 'Cholesterol lowering margarines' as this food product is acid forming and is not made with natural ingredients suitable for optimum health.

Beans – contain soluble fibre (pectin), helps reduce LDL. Pectin binds onto the cholesterol and eliminates it via the bowel. Look for natural bean foods, not tins of baked beans as these contain a lot of other unnecessary sauce, etc. Oats are good also. Celeriac, the vegetable, lowers cholesterol.

Garlic and Vitamin B3 – Garlic unsurpassed and helps to thin blood as well. Vitamin B3(niacin) also lowers LDL, with PRECAUTION on dosage.

Herbal Bitters – Digestive bitter tonics like dandelion, globe artichoke and milk thistle

Charcoal and Spirulina – 30g of activated charcoal 3 times a day can lower LDL levels by 40%. Do not take for extended periods of time. Spirulina has shown promising benefits also. Walnuts help reduce cholesterol

Avocados – contain phytochemicals called beta-sitosterols that reduce the absorption of cholesterol from foods. (these chemicals are widely used in the manufacture of cholesterol lowering drugs

Naturally occurring plant sterols reduce cholesterol levels.

Plant sterols found in natural foods are the leading weapons against high cholesterol and heart disease. These substances can reduce cholesterol by a minimum 10% if consumed regularly.
Plant sterols are an essential part of the cell structure of wood pulp, leaves, nuts, legumes, seeds, cereals, oils and many other foods. Plant sterols compete with the cholesterol in the gut and help prevent cholesterol from being absorbed.

It is important to eliminate the cause; it is no good trying to fix this unbalance if you don't address the cause. If you are consuming something that is contributing to your cholesterol level then you need to eliminate this first. Ensure sufficient fibre in your diet as this will slow down the absorption process in your digestive tract.

Chronic Diseases

Seen where there is excess toxins in the body and is a metabolic deficiency pattern.
Many tribal people around the globe do not get chronic disease like westerners do. Hunza tribal people of Pakistan is an example another is the Valcabambans of Ecuador.

We need more guidance and understanding so we can take more responsibility for our own health – we need educating so generations to come do not have prevalent health problems.

Circulation

To improve take Ginger, Nettle, Vitamin C, E, eliminate coffee altogether, quit smoking if you smoke.

What else can you do?

Exercise regularly. Please incorporate a little more than walking in your exercise routine – brisk walking not striding is more beneficial. You can get further information from your local fitness centre, or health worker. Massage, Shiatsu and Tai Chi are effective forms to stimulate circulation.

Aromatherapy - lavender, black pepper, rosemary are good. You can apply them directly or use diluted in carrier oil like linseed, apricot, olive, etc.

Foods to assist circulation include chilli, onions, turmeric and grapes.

Chest infection

Several areas need addressing;
1. Bowels need to be free and moving, so include sufficient fibre.
2. Improve digestion (and absorption) through prebiotic foods, especially Allium family of vegetables Garlic, onions, leeks, etc. Also, digestive enzymes like bromelain in pineapples are excellent.
3. Improve circulation internally, using garlic, ginger, chilli daily.
4. Light exercising to improve cardiovascular and airways circulation.
5. Do not chill your back from excess cold.
6. Sage tea taken hot. Several cups at a time will help stimulate circulation and is antibacterial.
7. Sufficient doses of Vitamin C and further supplementation of key vitamins and minerals.

Coffee / Caffeine products

These are no good as they leach calcium out of the body - one of the main problems with coffee. If you have coffee then use mainly fresh ground coffee – once you have tried the REAL thing you will not go back to instant coffee. Replace with herbal drinks; dandelion tea, carob. Brewed coffee is far better than instant coffee. If you have coffee try limit to three per day!

Colds

(Hint - Starve the cold – eat less foods. Consume herbal drinks, water, and remedies mentioned below.)

Freshly grated ginger in an infusion can clear up a cold. Sage and Garlic are good as is Cayenne pepper, (EXCELLENT). Cayenne pepper assists sweating and circulation and is a safe stimulant! Take 2 or 3 cups of hot sage at intervals to activate the body, produce strong circulation and throw off the infection.

Sore throat; take Sage and Thyme together steeped in a tea. Coughs then use herbs like; Thyme, Wood Betony, Marshmallow.

Remedy for persistent colds

Need to;
- cleanse the bowel (see section on bowels and digestion)
- Strengthen the immune system – this is so important!

Deep-seated chest problems try Thyme.
Insufficient Vitamin A foods in intake linked with decreased resistance to pneumonia.

Recurring colds, influenza, etc

1. <u>Your immune system is weak.</u> You need to strengthen your immune system so as to stave off illnesses.
2. Digestive system is compromised – you need to have clean bowels and wholesome foods. (See intestinal transit time for more information).

3. Body is acidic – you need to apply 80/20 rule. That is consume natural raw foods and alkalising foods 80% of the time. Keep intake of acid forming foods below 20% of your diet.
4. Stress has a major impact on our health. You need to talk with someone, work colleague, family member or friend for some input into your situation.

Constipation
Causes
Hint: Over-indulgence in meats, not sufficient fluids and not sufficient fruits and vegetables in our diet.
(See also Bowel section; Intestinal Transit Time.)

Remedy

Increase fibre intake - <u>do not allow body to re-absorb toxins via constipation.</u> You must have between 1 and 3 bowel movements a day. Linseed and olive oils can help.
Fresh fruit and vegetables, especially pears and apples. Try dandelion or bitters to further stimulate peristalsis of digestive system. Major improvements in spirits, energy, thinking and concentration can be expected when constipation is addressed. Prunes, dates, currants, apples, pears, cascara, plums, liquorice herb and many others all help.
Law of signatures; Black foods to remove [black] waste from the bowels. For example; prunes or raisins (black), help to cleanse and remove (black) waste from the intestines. Nature provides some answers to our health dilemmas in so much as; what we see in nature and foods, we see that they mimic our bodies.

Celiac Disease
Is the reaction to gluten, the protein of wheat and rye, oats and barley. Causes tissue changes in the mucosal cells of the duodenum. Symptoms include; loss of weight, distension of the abdomen and steatorrhea, (fat in the stools).

Remedy – Remove gluten foods from the diet; eat sufficient fresh fruit and vegetables, dried fruit, nuts (no peanuts), and legumes.

Cells of the body

The cells of our bodies have a finite thin layer of fat around them – similar analogy as the atmosphere envelopes earth. Now this layer of fat has to be the right fat so as to; let good nutrients in and allow the removal of cellular waste. If this coating of the cells is not correct then the cell does not function correctly and illnesses can develop. If the fat layer is a trans fat, (which is a bad fat used in many processed foods which solidifies when at room temperature), then this fat does not let in good nutrients nor allow the waste out. This is a basic explanation of how the cells work and I hope you can see the point that I am making regarding good and bad nutrition. To help your cells perform this process correctly you can see, now, why it is important to eat correctly and to understand how you are being affected by the foods you eat.

Cramps

Leg Cramps: Sign of lack of HCL (and other enzymes in the stomach), and / or Magnesium. Check circulation with your doctor – this is very important to ensure your heart and blood vessels are healthy and not clogged, etc. Consider improving your health now!

Cravings for chocolate

This may be a sign of Magnesium deficiency, because chocolate is high in Magnesium. The body can tell you that it is deficient in an element but not be exact in telling you which one this is – that is the problem. Best to consult with a qualified health practitioner than to overindulge in excess chocolate – don't you think?

Crohn's Disease See bowel section.

Also, drink one to two litres of PURE fresh water each day – a must! Supplements you can choose are Vitamin C, 2,000 – 4,000 mg per day, powder only. Zinc, 30 – 45 mg per day, and Linseed Oil, one tablespoon per day of raw and <u>fresh as possible</u>. Try to find the manufactured date on the container and purchase <u>refrigerated</u> linseed oil only as it tends to lose its potency if left in the light and at room temperature. Take lemon juice, ginger or other foods that will stimulate the release of digestive enzymes and improve this area that is often neglected.

Chronic Fatigue Syndrome – (See bowel section)

Dairy Products

(Hint – Only humans think they need the milk of another species to be healthy!)

The calcium in dairy products is altered causing it to be unsuitable for humans to consume. It is altered by pasteurization and homogenization and is turned into a hard mineral. Remember - cow's milk is for cows! Replace it with coconut milk, soy or, try it without any milk - your body will thank you! The body cannot use this denatured form correctly; it is then deposited inside the blood vessels. Powdered milk is hazardous also. Often oxidized cholesterol is added, creating a buildup of plaque in the arteries. Those countries that consume little milk, have little osteoporosis - I rest my case! Dairy products primarily affect the human glands, especially the reproductive glands, breast, uterus, thyroid, prostate, etc. Calcium is more readily assimilated from vegetable forms than from dairy products. You get your Calcium mostly from vegetables such as; broccoli and all cruciferous vegetables, oranges and others.

Dairy and allergies

An allergy to cow's milk in babies is not recognized so well. A colicky bottle-fed baby usually has a milk allergy. Also seen in babies as; recurrent croup, a dry cough and <u>ear blockages</u>. Also seen in Asthmatics, rhinitis, mucous in the nose, diarrhea, hives and eczema.

Alternatives to getting your Calcium

Of the vegetables then most all greens, especially Spinach, and including Parsley, Broccoli, and Kale. Sea vegetables are recommended as are legumes.

Of the nut family I find these are good sources of Calcium; Brazil nuts, Almonds, Sesame seeds, Sunflower seeds.

Dental – (see section on Teeth).

Diabetes

Non Insulin Dependent Diabetes Mellitus (NIDDM) is not influenced by genetics but has a cause in environmental factors which the main one is *lifestyle, overeating, obesity lack of exercise and incorrect nutrition.* Diabetics have lower levels of antioxidants. Body deficient in Chromium and Vanadium – two key minerals required in diabetic sufferers.

Remedy

Addressing your diet and including exercise is the key to the treatment regime. You must also remove the foods that accentuate diabetes.

Supplements include; Magnesium (Always deficient in Diabetics, without it you can develop retinopathy), Vitamin C (this is a strong antioxidant, helps prevent tissue damage in the cells), Vitamin E (improves insulin resistance and has protective effect on the oxidation of LDL Cholesterol), Chromium and the B Vitamin group all help. Alpha-Lipoic acid (ALA), may relieve numbness or burning sensation in feet and fingers that is a common side effect of diabetes and may reverse the nerve damage. The nutrient has strong anti-oxidant properties, improves cellular energy production and supports detoxification. ALA doesn't affect blood glucose, so is safe for diabetics. Supplements available.

See your health practitioner for suggestions and advice.

Magnesium

Diabetics are deficient in Magnesium as they lose it via their kidneys. Hence, diabetics are prone to developing retinopathy due to this contributing factor – and when supplemented the retinopathy improves.

Vitamin C
Vitamin C prevents conversion of sugar into sorbitol within the cell, therefore, is important in preventing tissue damage.

Vitamin E
Improves insulin resistance, has protective effect on the oxidization of LDL cholesterol.

B complex, beta-carotene, bioflavanoids, zinc and selenium are important antioxidants and assist the enzymatic processes.

Diet and Nutrition
One of the most important points in our health is the food we consume.
Dr. Bernard Jensen, Naturopath and Iridologist once said;
We must take care of 3 things;
"BRAIN (thoughts), BOWEL (king) and the NERVOUS SYSTEM."
The foods we consume must be of optimum nutritional value, avoid processed foods, additives, preservatives, colourings and denatured foods devoid of nutritional value – Do not compromise your health! How can the blood supply pure nutrients to all the cells when all that is circulating is a contaminated blood supply? Degenerative processes are prone to take hold – demand the best. Demand to know what is in the food you buy from the supermarket and other sources. Take aways and coloured drinks are a no-no, as is white bread to name but a few. Don't expect the liver to cope with all the below average supply of nutrients.
Ill health situations may not show up for years, but reflect on your health now so that in the future you will add years to your life and be much healthier.
A misunderstood approach to dieting exists in western societies: The misconception with western style approaches to dieting is to stop eating. This is not the correct way of dealing with weight management. Eat correct proportions of the correct food, (as natural as you can find and preferably uncooked.) The secret to longevity is a slightly empty

stomach! If you eat until you are exactly full then the digestive process is working overtime, and stresses the body's internal balance.

Digestion / Indigestion
Remedy

Low acid producing foods, fresh fruit and vegetables, fibre foods and try the herbs ginger and liquorice.
Take Hydrochloric acid (HCl) tablets to find out if you have low or high stomach acid. In most cases it will be low stomach acid balance that is causing problems, not high acid content. Trialing HCl tablets are completely safe and anyone can do this simple test. It is safe, but please check with your Natural Therapist or other health practitioner for further advice.
Do not take antacid preparations, especially those with aluminium-based ingredients. If symptoms persist seek advice from a relevant practitioner.

For low level of HCl in the stomach you can take a tablespoon of Apple Cider Vinegar in a glass of water half an hour before meals.

Symptoms of low acid in the stomach can include anemia, low energy and leg cramps.
To assist digestion,
1. Identify cause (Eliminate known offenders, see diet section.)
2. Bitters to stimulate, Swedish bitters, Gentian and Wormwood, (before meals.)
3. Lemon juice / Cider Vinegar, ginger or vitamin C containing foods.
4. Digestive enzymes - papain, bromelain, and probiotics like yoghurt. (friendly bacteria.)

How do you know if your digestive system is absorbing the nutrients? Your Naturopath or Iridologist can tell you. The greyish, brown signs that an Iridologist can see in the digestive tract area of your eye usually means the body is not capable of absorbing good food.

Sluggish digestive systems require fast acting iron foods to burn out rubbish. Garlic, fenugreek and leafy green vegetables (RAW).

Acute digestive disturbances you can try Slippery Elm.

Elevated pH levels in the stomach interfere with protein digestion permitting bacterial overgrowth. Proteins are not, then, broken down correctly and result in toxifying the system.

Improving digestion

Health starts with correct digestion of foods. Likened to a smoldering pile of newspapers on a fire do not burn and produce acrid smoke and waste so does our digestive system if foods are not correctly digested: Without correct digestion we will not be supplying our bodies with the essential nutrients it NEEDS! If you are unsure check with your local health practitioner versed in nutrition and digestive function – you will be glad you did! Probably the most vital aspect of regenerating health is a good source of digestive enzymes. Digestive enzymes break down our food and nutrients as they enter the body and allow us to absorb assimilate those nutrients. Again, most people are deficient in digestive enzymes, and the body will not heal without a sufficient supply. Deficiency of digestive enzymes places an incredible burden on the pancreas which depletes our system.

Digestion – Low stomach acid and absorption signs

1. Eliminate known cause
2. HCL tablets trial to test for low acid production
3. Bitter foods to stimulate secretion; Turmeric, Lemon juice, Ginger, Licorice, Apple Cider Vinegar
4. Digestion assisting enzymes – Bromelain (pineapples), papain (paw paw), yoghurt

Malabsorption Signs
- Fingernail strength test for nutritional deficiencies (cracked, peeling, weak)
- Low energy
- Recurring illnesses and low immunity

- Arthritis type ailments – poor digestion and malabsorption of vits. And mins. And lack of enzymes
- Leg cramps (esp over 50's showing poor assimilation of Ca, Mg, K and others
- Dilated blood vessels in the cheeks
- Food allergies
- Bloating, belching, flatulence
- Acne and other skin disorders
- Undigested food in the stools
- Indigestion, diarrhea, constipation
- Headaches

Foods that help

Garlic, red onions, celery, radish, pumpkin, green vegetables, BEETROOT, linseed oil, Turmeric (also anti-cancer), milk thistle, wormwood.

Further notes....

- Low stomach acid conditions greatly contribute to nutritional deficiencies,
- Elevated PH interferes with protein digestion – permitting bacterial overgrowth, resulting in toxification of the system.
- Rheumatoid Arthritis and little no gastric acid (hypochlorhydria), go hand in hand. RA – check bacterial overgrowth in gut. As we get older our stomach's produce less acid and pepsin – this inefficiency is often accompanied with gas.
- Can be a sign of 'Progressive Stomach Failure'
- Ulcers are caused by disruption to the protective barrier(mucous/bicarbonate) of the stomach – Helicobacter Pylori is most often the cause. You will note someone with extreme and pungent breath.
- Poor protein digestion can lead to food allergies.

- Antacid preparations reduce acidity and increase the risk of pathogens colonizing especially in the intestinal tract.
- Intragastric pH value of stomach is less than 4, <u>acid suppressing drugs drive pH greater than 5</u>, allowing bacteria to thrive

You need a strong acid barrier!

Low stomach acid conditions greatly contribute to nutritional deficiencies, EVEN IF YOU EAT CORRECTLY!

Some health signs linked to poor digestion – Skin problems, acne, headaches, low on energy, fatigue, anemia.

Low Acid – What to do.
1. Eliminate cause
2. Bitters to stimulate. Try raw Ginger as this is a good digestive tonic
3. Lemon juice or cider vinegar
4. Digestive enzymes, Bromelain (Pineapples), Papain (Paw Paw) + Vitamin B12
5. Test stomach acid level (can use hair analysis for iron, calcium, zinc levels. An accurate pH test may be needed
6. Test for serious gastric / oesophageal disease if not, continue with natural approach
7. Can further test stomach acid levels with HCL / pepsin capsules. Take with meals.
8. Use probiotics (friendly bacteria, Lactobacillus, etc.)

If chronic, or strong pain then have GP check;
- pH of stomach
- Test for atrophic gastritis
- Helicobacter Pylori infection (more common than you think)
- Vitamin / Mineral malabsorption
- Other problems

Signs of Low Acid

Heartburn, indigestion, gas, discomfort in the stomach area. Resist antacid medication if possible.

Finger nail strength test for nutritional deficiencies (cracked, peeling, soft.) Leg cramps (especially over 50's) sign of inadequate digestion and assimilation of Calcium, Magnesium and Potassium, (and other minerals). Pepsin (required for digestion in the stomach)cannot be formed at pH5 or greater (needed for protein assimilation) Lack of HCL in stomach symptoms can be; Anemia, low energy, etc.

Acid base required for stomach, then the chyme (food) moves into the small intestines which are strongly alkaline. Low stomach acid conditions contribute greatly to nutritional deficiencies, even if you eat correctly. Correct acidic environment then assists in solubility of Iron, Calcium, Zinc, etc. The digestive system is KING. Proper digestion of foods, including proteins, carbohydrates, fats, vitamins, minerals and all important enzymes, is essential to maintain and fuel the whole body. By supplying good nutrition, via good digestion, we assist in strengthening the immune system, thereby reducing the opportunities of pathogens, viruses and cell altering diseases (cancers), taking hold!

Foods that assist digestion

Chickpeas are excellent. The Alliam family; onions, chives, garlic. Fruits and vegetables in general help including pineapples, Paw Paw and mangoes.

Bitter foods help stimulate the digestive process – Dandelion, Ginger, Peppermint, Wormwood, Milk Thistle, Globe Artichoke.

Herbal – Coriander, Mint, Tarragon, Ginger, TURMERIC, Capsicum. Acute digestive problems take Slippery Elm. A powder form is available from most health shops.

Low stomach acid signs;

- * Bloating, belching, flatulence
- * Dilated blood vessels in cheeks and nose
- * Indigestion, constipation, diarrhea
- * Iron deficiency

* Food allergies
* Undigested food in stools
* Skin problems
* Week, peeling, cracked fingernails
* Headaches
* <u>Leg cramps</u> (especially over 50 years of age), are signs of inadequate digestion and assimilation of Calcium, Magnesium and Potassium minerals.

Remedy

Low acid producing foods, fresh fruit and vegetables, fibre foods and try the herbs ginger and liquorice. Take Hydrochloric acid (HCl) tablets to find out if you have low or high stomach acid. In most cases it will be low stomach acid balance that is causing problems, not high acid content. Trialing HCl tablets are completely safe and anyone can do this simple test. It is safe, but please check with your Natural Therapist or other health practitioner for further advice.

Do not take antacid preparations, especially those with aluminium-based ingredients. If symptoms persist seek advice from a relevant practitioner.

Health of GI tract

Health of GI tract improved with foods rich in Vitamin B and rich in iron and phosphorous, eg. Prunes (black foods cure black waste in the body – nature's signature)

Prebiotics

Certain foods that have a special kind of carbohydrate that helps the 'good' bacteria grow and flourish by feeding them and keeping them healthy – so they can fight off 'bad' bacteria.

Prebiotic foods – Garlic (raw), Asparagus (lightly steamed or raw), Onions (red and brown), leeks (raw or lightly steamed), bananas (smaller benefit need 65 a day to get your quota)

(Note: I have mentioned lightly steamed as overcooking destroys the very key nutrients that are there to help you.) Prebiotic foods compliment probiotic foods (yoghurt).

Intestinal parasites
Chickpeas help to address stomach parasites.
Foods – **for the digestive enhancement process**

> Carrots, Lettuce, parsley, currants, broccoli, tomato, cucumber, radish, LEMONS, Garlic, sunflower seeds, other nuts (avoid peanuts), fresh fruit, GREEN LEAFY Vegetables (for folic acid), beetroot, silver beet (LIGHTL steamed), dates, prunes, celery, almonds, cabbage, brussels sprouts, pumpkin seeds.

Revise your pantry! Look at your pantry and eliminate foods that aren't natural. For example; pastry products remain in their hardened state – what do you think this does to your body? These thicken and harden our bodies – seen in our hardened and thickened arteries. See section on 'Human Intervention' or HI foods.
LEMON Water daily!

Depression
Seek help if you feel depressed for a period of time. Get your mind occupied with a passion, look deep, seek help from friends or someone you can trust with matters of the heart, go on a holiday meet new people. (See Depression in Section 2)

Diseases
Most all diseases are related to toxic substances in the body. These can include the wrong foods to consume like; processed foods, sugars, red meat, excess dairy products and last but not least, margarine! Diseases are related to an imbalance in the body.
Prevention of disease – Garlic, LEMON JUICE, dandelion and dandelion greens, blueberries. Take the juice of several lemons regularly,

diluted half with water. As with most diseases they usually take a fair time to develop even up to forty years before they show up.

Doctors

"The doctor of the future will give no medicines but will interest his or her patients in the care of the human frame, in diets and the cause and prevention of disease." (Thomas Edison.)

Doctors need to educate us on correct understanding of health. We need the support of Naturopaths, nutrition experts and the like to TRULY make a difference to our overall health – now! It is through this understanding that we will be encouraged to take action.

Doctrine of Signatures - *Seen in nature and foods that 'like cures like'*

For example: the Walnut's shape resembles that of the human brain, hence Walnuts are good for the brain. Prunes are 'black' in colour and are conducive to cleaning the bowels, (the 'black' waste of the body). This is not a coincidence it is fact of how effective nature is and how we should pay attention to what how nature can heal us. Beetroot is red and helps to support the blood and related organs!

Drugs

Recreational drugs cause an <u>alteration to the DNA chain at a cellular level</u>. They also reduce your motivation and drive in life – they affect your kidney energy strongly. Studies have shown a link to the development of Schizophrenia with Marijuana users.

Eczema

Linked with the elimination and circulation functions of the internal body. If the amount of toxins exceeds our body's abilities to eliminate, there is a build up in the blood.

Linked to the quality of the blood. There are toxins in the blood more likely caused by poor quality or incorrect foods and / or poor absorption through the digestive tract. Recommend you see a Naturopath or G.P. to confirm malabsorption of the digestive tract. The elimination and circulation function is compromised due to toxins and excess fat, sugars, refined foods and additives.

Remedy

Eliminate all major allergens esp. milk & dairy, eggs, peanuts, watch wheat. Eliminate salt and sugar! Limit animal products, fats, etc. Include 'fatty' fish such as salmon, herring or mackerel in the diet. (The good fats, Omega 3, EFA's found in Linseed, most nuts, etc.) Fruits and vegetables (raw), to 'clean out' the intestines and bowel and allow the body to heal itself. (See section on Bowels).

Topical
Aloe Vera unsurpassed as to the benefits. Fresh Aloe Vera leaf is best – commercial products tend to have other additives included.

Internal
Licorice (the herb) can be used safely with good results – anti-inflammatory and anti-allergenic effects. Aloe Vera is excellent internally, however, you need to be guided by your health practitioner.

Supplements
Quality multi vitamin and mineral is recommended. Eczema sufferers lack certain vits and minerals. Quality supplements from your local health practitioner, not the supermarket, is the best source.
Plenty of fluids and fresh fruit and vegs. – not processed or packaged foods.
Consult a reputable natural health practitioner – Naturopath, Chinese Medicine, Herbalist, Dietitian that is focused on natural foods to assist.

Elimination channels of the body
These are; bowels, kidneys, lungs, lymph and skin (and liver.)
All elimination channels must be functioning properly to assist the body.

Enzymes

An extremely important constituent of natural foods are the enzymes they contain. These enzymes are crucial for assisting many processes within the human body. We need the enzymes from plant foods!

Deficiency in enzymes: Seen when we process, cook or intervene with processing, these wonderful foods nature provides. You will not find as many essential enzymes in, for example, a meat pie as you would in a handful of fresh berries. Enzymes are essential for maintaining our health – I cannot overemphasize this! They are the switches if you like of many bodily processes and assist proteins to function correctly. It is the foundation of healthy bodies, without them you may age more rapidly.

Exercise

(Hint – Exercise is a CRITICAL part of lifestyle improvement, and has many benefits, so discipline yourself today!)

Without exercise the muscles atrophy and the cardiovascular system weakens. When the muscles are not active the vessels cannot pulsate and the blood will not circulate correctly. This lack of activity leads to a <u>stagnation of blood and body moisture, which</u> can lead to degeneration of tissue. Please include exercises with your weekly routine. Yoga, Tai Chi, Pilates, etc., are all very useful for ridding the body of congestion in the muscles, joints and digestive system. However, exercise has far reaching benefits, which includes the mind. Extremely important is the role of an exercise regime, however, most important is the need for resistance, or weight bearing, training. Swimming, walking, bicycle riding is good, but we need to include resistance exercises to take full benefit. Resistance exercises like; power walking, swimming, lifting weights. Something that involves the muscles more.

Note; *Muscles that are not used are abused, and this becomes a repository for toxins and fat.*

Women especially, need to include resistance training weekly at least. Your bones respond as well by becoming stronger and tend to retain their constitution a little more when we exercise regularly.

One essential key to staying young is exercise and building muscle.

Unlike fat, which is fairly inert, muscle is active tissue. <u>Blood runs through it, bringing in nutrients and carrying off waste</u>. Muscle tissue speeds up metabolism; the heart must pump a greater volume of blood to supply the muscles, food is digested more efficiently to get energy to the muscles. As we age and exercise less the <u>metabolism slows down accordingly</u> as there is not as much demand for nutrition supply for the muscles. The metabolism backs off a little and takes it easy. Building muscle keeps the metabolic fire burning among many other benefits. You have to find the muscle building exercise that helps you and you are comfortable to committing to this regime REGULARLY!

If you maintain exercise in your lifestyle then the muscles will not atrophy and the hormone building blocks will not decrease as fast.

Another benefit of muscle building exercise is that you can eat a little more and not put on weight – that's got to be a good benefit alone!

Eyes

Your eyes can show the health of your internal body function. Eye problems can be a sign that your body may have sub-clinical patterns taking place. In other words, your body is not functioning at its best, this in turn, may show as poor health in the future. Here, an Iridologist or a health professional experienced in reading the patterns and colours in the eyes, can offer some further guidance.

Twitching eyes take Magnesium Phosphate. For Magnesium eat plenty of green vegetables, (remember to lightly cook only if you have to), and nuts in your eating plan.

Cataracts – seen where partial blockage to the brain of arteries (Atherosclerosis).

You will usually see halos around lights if you have cataracts

Remedy.

Consume blueberries, and other berries. Blueberries help to inhibit the formation of cataracts. Avoid margarine! Margarines are acid forming foods and contain artificial products – they are toxic for the body. Chelated minerals needed to clean out the blood vessels of the body, remove toxins, excess cholesterol and plaque from the artery walls.

Blood vessel disorders of the eyes, especially diabetes, may respond to bioflavonoid and/or Vitamin C treatment.

Vitamin A deficiency,
1. Night blindness
2. Slow recovery from bright lights – especially car headlights.

Zinc is required for the enzyme that activates Vitamin A in the visual process. This deficiency can result in 'night blindness'.

Dark area below eyes can show; lack of sleep, exhausted kidneys, or low iron intake or absorption.

Bulging Eyes – sign of goiter or problem with Thyroid function.

Pale flesh on inner eyelid – indication of anemia. Need plenty of green vegetables, raisins, broccoli, etc. and combine with increase Vitamin C powder to aid absorption of iron better.

Bags under the eyes – is a sign of Kidney function and fluid balance in the body. If you see puffy eye bags then there is excess fluid in the body. This can also indicate the efficiency of your bowels. Pay attention to this sign.

Glaucoma

Is where the optic nerve at the back of the eye is slowly destroyed, resulting in progressive loss of vision. It is seen with a build-up of pressure in the eye. Symptoms include;

Blurred vision, apparent coloured rings around lights, loss of side vision, and pain and redness of the eye.

Have eyes tested regularly over 40 yrs of age. Why? The eyes can be an early detection system of future illnesses and diseases. Please see your Naturopath or professional versed in Iridology as they can help you in this area. Reduce oxidation and pressure in the eye area. Antioxidant foods beneficial and include all coloured vegetables. Grape seed extract is good, as is ginkgo biloba and bilberry. Exercise along with improved nutrition is so important to slow down and reverse glaucoma, (and other eye problems).

The white areas of the eyes

- Blue: If the whites of your eyes appear blue can be a sign of Osteoporosis (lack of Calcium).
- Yellow: sign of liver problems as in jaundice
- Red: indicates infection or high blood pressure (if seen without prominent blood vessels). And is a sign of under functioning liver.
- Red blotches on the whites of the eye are usually a sign of high blood pressure.

Laser surgery may be considered if badly deteriorated.

Macular Degeneration

This is becoming an ever-increasing eye complaint. As I have said before that the eyes are the window to how your body is operating internally. There seems to be poor nutrition and excess waste in the body that is being seen as deteriorated vision.

Remedy

Remove processed foods, salt, sugar, pastries from your diet. (Refer to acid/alkaline balance section for more information.) We need to reduce free radical damage to the body that is also showing up as deteriorated eye sight.
- Take antioxidants, especially grape seed extract.
- Consume more fruit and vegetables in their natural state, especially all types of berries.
- Eliminate acid producing foods (fast foods, processed foods, margarine and heavy red meats.
- Stop smoking if you are a smoker and curb alcohol intake to a sensible level.

(A point worth mentioning; atherosclerosis is almost always seen in macular degeneration cases).

Face

Petechial hemorrhages (tiny visible blood vessels), around the face can be a sign of depleted Vitamin C. Take this as a high dose powder with bioflavonoids which help capillaries and the absorption of Vitamin C.

Fasting

1 day fast and cleanse plan!
1 day fasting, consuming pure water and herbal teas as required. Following day start with lemon juice and yoghurt, then gradually return to a healthy diet, of fresh fruit and vegetables, nuts, grains and juices. (Sorry, no take away, processed foods, etc.) If constipated try prunes / prune juice, pears, apples, leafy green vegetables and senna pod herbal tea, until bowels move.

Option

Fasting one day a week, or several days a month at a time consuming one food item. For example; grapes only, brown rice only are some foods that are beneficial. So you can consume as much as you want of the chosen food for the day. This is a more tolerable format to help cleanse your body without the stress of not eating anything. You may wish to put aside a day, (or several days), to do this. I know some people like to try this on your holidays, consuming one food for the day and having herbal drinks or just plain water – your body will thank you for it!

Food

(Hint - the earth is covered by 70% water, our bodies are 70% water, and vegetables are mostly 70% water. We can see that consuming more vegetables would be more harmonious and suitable for our bodies – don't you think?)

If you have plans for the future which do not include nagging illnesses, dangerous medicines, hospitals and untimely death, then consume a large proportion of your food **RAW**, as nature intended. Cooking kills enzymes in food. Most vitamin and mineral supplements do not contain natural enzymes as nature intended <u>and cannot, altogether, compensate</u> for the natural approach to food consumption. However, there are times in which some vitamin supplements can be of benefit. Avoid sugar as it leaches the body of precious minerals and vitamins, and produces an over-acid condition.

HI (Human Intervention) **versus GI** (Glycaemic index) foods
Don't be as concerned so much about 'GI' foods; we should be concerned about 'HI' foods. When we process natural foods more we lose valuable nutrients and enzymes that are the very thing that supports our function. It is this human intervention in natural foods that has an impact on our health.

The more humans alter the food the more this contributes to our poor health!

Processed foods - contain any of the following;

> Emulsifiers, preservatives, dyes, artificial flavours and sweeteners, humuctants, bleaches, neutralisers, disinfectants, thickeners, anti-foaming and anti-caking agents, hydrolisers, deodorants, hydrogenators, sulfites, fumigants, stabilisers, antibiotics, steroids, growth hormones and irradiation. *And you thought you were eating FOOD!*

Food Allergies

Poor protein absorption can lead to food allergies – have digestion checked by your health professional, as low stomach secretions, (and poor digestion), can adversely affect the assimilation of proteins, among other nutrients.

Also, consuming incorrect foods has an effect. (See section on digestion.)

Food Labeling

Always read the labels on packaged foods. Food companies can call their bread 'Whole meal' but may only contain a small percentage of the flour as true wholegrain – the rest could be processed white flour. White flour that has been processed contains minimal nutrients as they are removed during the milling phase. (Can you see now, how we can consume foods and yet some [a lot] may not be supporting us, nutritionally?)

Some fruits and vegetables that are treated in some way include;

Onions – often treated to stop them sprouting, or shooting. (If they shoot they are still alive)

Imported garlic can be fumigated with a toxic process to stop unwanted bacteria, etc

Potatoes – often crops are sprayed upon maturity to kill the potato tops so as to get them to the supermarket sooner.

Ensure you wash vegetables, especially broccoli, and celery – wash in warm water.

Cooking Oils

Sunflower, Canola oils, and some other oils used in food preparation, are hydrogenated to thicken and harden them, thereby keeping the food they are in thick and hard – a commercial packet of biscuits, pastry foods etc. Check the processed foods you buy. Some foods do not contain these oils.

> What do you think these thickened and hardened foods we consume are doing to our bodies? They are lining our blood vessels and 'coating' the cells of our body. This coating on the cells hinders the natural cleansing and delivery of nutrients to the cells – the very things we need to help preserve our health!

Fruit

Hint: Fruits cleanse the body internally, vegetables heal!

Consuming fruits in their natural state is essential. The reason is; fruits cleanse the body of waste and toxins. Citrus fruits, in particular, contain bioflavonoids, in the pith. The pith is the white part of oranges and lemons, for example, and this compound helps support our blood vessels as well. Fruit does not put weight on yet assists the cleansing of the digestive system amongst many other benefits.

Gall Bladder (See also Liver)

Consume apples, 2 to 5 apples, a day *

Apples stimulate the secretion of digestive juices and aid protein absorption. (You need a good digestive process to assist the body processes and help soften and eliminate gall stones).
They contain pectin, which binds to cholesterol and helps soften stones and then is excreted from the body. They aid in the elimination of uric acid (as seen in gout conditions), and help to ease constipation and keep the bowels clean.
DOSAGE: Take as many as you want. 2-5 apples a day will greatly assist your condition.
(Note: I have many comments of the personal health benefits gained from this food). Also, fresh apple juice taken daily not commercial juice that is processed with sugars! These products are really a waste of time.

Try a cup of grated beetroot and carrot taken with juice of a lemon and grated apple or add chopped cucumber. Take your combination daily (or at least every two days) for 1 week, then at least every second day for another 3 weeks. Beetroot is labelled the, 'Vitality plant'.

Point to consider

Reviewing the foods you consume will greatly benefit your condition and can help to reduce symptoms to a minimum. We need to reduce acid forming foods, (these are known to cause irritation in the body), and replace with alkaline producing foods. These will help supply better nutrition to the cells of the body.

Other Key Healing Foods

Linseed oil, quality olive and grape seed oil, fish, grapes, cherries, berries, cabbage (raw if possible), beans, onion family, cucumbers, LOTS OF GREEN LEAFY VEGETABLES!
Red-blue berries; Cherries, hawthorn berries, blueberries and others are rich sources of anthocyanidins and procyanidins
Fruits and vegetables supply the balance of nutrients and enzymes for the body to maintain correct function. Keep in mind – Fruits cleanse the body, vegetables heal and fortify the body!

Note: You must eliminate those 'problem' foods that are known to aggravate your condition.
<u>You cannot make healthy changes to your diet if you still consume the problem foods.</u>

> **AVOID** – Fatty foods, chops and sausages, pastries, cakes, sugar, salt, sweets, cut down on dairy products, <u>protein drinks</u>, etc.

Eliminate the following acid forming foods

Margarine, sugar, chops, sausages and watch out for the 'bad' fats in pastry foods, in sweet biscuits, pies and pasties, pizzas, etc.

What do these fats do to us?

These fats, at a cellular level, coat the cells of the body with a 'hard' layer and <u>do not allow correct transfer of nutrients into the cells and allow efficient elimination of waste from the cells</u>. (Just like any living thing, cells of the body need to be supplied with the correct nutrients to operate efficiently).

Bile production helps to rid intestines of microorganisms. To increase bile flow production naturally, you can take Choline (1000mg) and Methionine (500mg) daily.

Signs to watch

Brown patches on the back of your hand can indicate dysfunction of the Liver / Gall Bladder, along with pains under the ribs on the RIGHT SIDE.

General Food Tonics for the Body

> Ginger – Garlic – Sage – Wheat grass juice (all are excellent!)
> Chilli, Cayenne Pepper – the all time stimulant for the body!

Genes

Genes can be influenced by lifestyle and dietary factors. For example; a large study was conducted in Canada in which 27,000 people consumed a diet of raw fruit and vegetables to overcome the effects of genes that increase the risk of heart disease. The researchers found a reduction in heart problems. I strongly believe that nutrition, at a cellular level, can influence genes more than we care to think.

Genetics

You can strengthen your genes. Yes it is possible!

The only thing genetic about an illness is poor diet advice –food for thought!

Centuries ago Scurvy was considered a genetic illness until they found that the diet of sailors was deficient in Vitamin C.

Breast cancer in women can sometimes be labelled as genetic when in fact, the lifestyle factors, including principles of nutrition, are followed through the generations.

Remedy

DHEA Enhancement plan (Natural form);
1. Regular exercise
2. Stress management
3. Contentment
4. Adequate sleep
5. Relaxation (and meditation) at least once a day
6. Weight Loss
7. Nutritional supplementation – A, B2, B6, B12, C, E, zinc, magnesium, Folic acid, TMG (Trymethylglycine)
8. Vitamin C 2000mg per day, (and methyl sulfonylmethane 750-1000mg daily and can supplement with amino acids Tyrosine and Phophotidylserine P.S.
9. Herbs such as Ginseng and Licorice
10. <u>Consume wholesome, natural fruits, vegetables, nuts and grains</u>. Keep away from processed foods, especially bad fats found in these.

What you eat and how you live literally changes your genes.

Glands
Adrenal

These small glands situated on the top of the kidneys have such a powerful role to play. They produce adrenalin among other chemicals. These glands are programmed into the circadian rhythm, so that a burst of these energizing hormones first thing in the morning helps us to start the day. If you do not feel alive in the mornings then re-address your health.

Remedy

Improve your diet, stop smoking, remove the stress and see a Natural Therapist or similar, for further advice.
Take Vitamin C, B5, E and choline, magnesium and essential fatty acids. No, your hamburger does not contain such a thing. Try foods like; sunflower, sesame seeds, nuts, olives, grape seed oil, avocadoes and fish.

Pancreas

Pancreatic enzymes assist in ridding of microorganisms from the intestines. Herbs that support the pancreas without disturbing blood sugar levels are; Cinnamon, nutmeg, fennel, celery and aniseed, kelp and alfalfa, liquorice and chamomile tea.

For hypoglycaemia (low blood sugar), eat a little and often. See your Natural Therapist or doctor if symptoms persist. Metaphysical link; the Pancreas is the balance organ - are you out of balance?

Thyroid

Signs of dysfunction include;
Hypo-function - weight gain, feeling excessively cold, fluid retention, fatigue, dry hair, constipation, drooping eyelids and need for sleep. Some may have a persistent sore throat.
Hyper-function - Speedy individual, lean type of person.
Kelp is excellent for rebalancing the thyroid gland.

Lymph

If your lymph glands are swollen then, most likely, the body is fighting some pathogenic situation or illness. This is where many immune cells attack pathogens and bad bugs. You need to see a health professional to look further into the problem.

Prostate problems

Eliminate coffee, tea, alcohol and sugar.

Remedy

The herb Saw Palmetto is excellent (160mg twice a day), Zinc and Selenium from Pumpkin seeds and other nuts, Silica tablets, and tomatoes support the prostate. You can also use Linseed oil under 4 months old, Nettle (especially nettle root extract), Raspberry leaf Tea and unprocessed natural foods. Any drugs, including antihistamines, can turn a partly obstructed prostate into a fully obstructed one. Parsnips are a good source of Bromine which is excellent for the glands. Have your health practitioner check you for inflammation patterns in the body – this can be done with a simple blood test (see section on tests). Have yourself checked regularly as early detection is important.

Gout

Seen as the overproduction of uric acid coming from purine foods, (nucleoproteins found especially in glandular meats), and yeast, fats and refined carbohydrates. When not excreted they build up in joints, crystallizing especially in the big toe. Alcohol inhibits secretion of uric acid from the kidneys.

Remedy

Omit organ meats, heavy red meats, sardines. Eat asparagus, beans, cabbage, lentils, peas and spinach. Dark berries for proanthocyanidin(antioxidant), content Consuming cherries, blueberries, or cranberries and drinking celery seed tea daily can lower uric acid waste. Rolled oats, asparagus, dandelion and most salad vegetables are good also. Drink sufficient clean water to help flush toxins from the body. Eliminate sugars from the diet, replace with honey. (See also the section on Kidneys.)

Hair

Hair condition is an indication of liver, kidney and sex organ health.
Split ends - excess yin foods like processed foods, fats, dairy products and red meats.
Brittle - excess salt / animal foods damaging kidney energy. Include more natural vegetable intake to ensure good mineral balance.
Grey hair - excess stress and salt. (These both harm the kidneys.) Lacking Zinc or Folic acid.
Dandruff - incorrect foods being consumed. Think what you ate in the time preceding dandruff appearing. Outside hair indicates inside hair condition. (i.e.; the micro hairs like cilia in the intestines and lungs.)

Hay fever

This is an allergic condition of the mucous membranes of the eyes, ears and nose.

Remedy

REMOVE dairy products totally! Raw garlic, parsley and fenugreek. Ensure bowels are moving freely. A cleanse may be needed to move out old waste that may have accumulated. Minerals like; Magnesium Phosphate, Sodium Chloride and Silica can address hay fever as well, your health shop can help here. Address your diet – consult your Naturopath.

Headaches

Can be many causes and here are a few suggestions that work the best.
Stress type headache - take hot bath with calming oils like lavender, chamomile, juniper and orange. Massage, or other physical therapies are

very effective. Most of all find the cause and fix it - do not compromise your health, headaches if they continue are a sign of some other problem. Lemon or lavender on forehead and temples can help.

Migraine types – Magnesium supplementation can help. You will need to check with your health practitioner. General types - take high dose Vitamin C powder, a glass or two of water and go for a brisk run or bike ride. Hangover types - drink a couple of glasses of cool, clean water and go for a brisk run or bike ride. Yes, this works well and you will find your headache has gone by the time you get home. Try it!

Herbs like Feverfew, Sage, and Wood Betony are good. Check for poor digestion, your natural therapist can help.

Foods that help are Walnuts, chickpeas, and wheat germ as these contain the amino acid Tryptophan that helps with calming the body. Eliminate hard cheeses, bacon, ham, yeast extracts, and CHOCOLATE. There are other foods to watch, however, these are the most common. If pain persists or is extreme, seek medical advice.

Health

Don't expect to take a pill, vitamin tablet or eat a healthier food if the majority of your food you eat are contributing to health problems – a little of a good thing will not fix a big health problem.

You are being affected by the foods you eat, and,
The foods you are not eating!

Heart

Heart Attack modification program; Diet modification, Omega 3 oils, a happy heart!

One sign of a disposition towards cardiovascular problems; diagonal earlobe crease seen on the bottom of ear lobe.

Check with your local practitioner before self-diagnosing.

Conventional Heart risk factors;
- ➢ High intake of saturated fat
- ➢ High Cholesterol
- ➢ Smoking
- ➢ Hypertension

- Family history
- Diabetes
- Obesity
- Alcohol
- Sedentary lifestyle

Modern heart risk factors;
- Oxidised LDL
- Eicasinoids
- Homocysteine
- Inflammation
- Lipoprotein-a
- Fibrinogen
- Syndrome-X
- Unresolved stress

Blood tests recommended for Cardiovascular Care.

Stop accumulation of plaque on arterial walls – take antioxidants, Vitamin C, green tea, garlic.

Damage is caused by Heterocyclic amines the by-products of deep frying, barbecuing, or grilling something. Especially seen in well cooked meats like hamburgers and take away foods.

The body tries to repair the damaged blood vessel wall, and if the immune system is not strong the body will not be able to repair itself correctly. The lesions remain partially unhealed, and plaque starts to build up on them.

Crease on Earlobe.

People with a diagonal crease on the earlobe are more prone to heart disease. The crease doesn't cause heart disease, however, this is generally a sign of increased risk. What should you do? Pay particular attention to your heart health.

Vitamins for the heart

Selenium helps protect against heart disease. <u>Co Q10 is essential.</u> Minerals needed are Calcium, Potassium and Magnesium. These are the main mineral requirements for the heart.

Formation of coronary artery lesions (atheroma)
- Low-density lipoproteins (LDL) in blood plasma
- LDL infiltration into artery wall
- Oxidation of LDL by activated oxygen species, catalyzed by iron and/or copper complexes
- Alternatively, pre-formed oxidized LDL from diet can infiltrate artery wall
- Formation of foam cells
- Injury to artery walls
- Adherence of blood platelets

Take Lecithin, Vitamin C, Garlic, Omega 3, Gingko Biloba, *(Contraindication; overdose can lower BP via thinning of the blood.)*
Meditation, relaxation and stress release go hand in hand with a healthy heart.

Research today finds that oxidative stress, due to inflammations from nutritional and environmental hazards, is the primary cause of cancer, Alzheimer's disease, Parkinson's disease, arthritis and all forms of heart disease. An example; heterocyclic amines are the by-products of deep frying, barbecuing, or grilling something. Well cooked meat is loaded with heterocyclic amines. These are extremely destructive. When you eat a hamburger, those heterocyclic amines are released into your system. Then they cause damage to the arterial walls. The body tries to repair this damage, but if the immune system is not strong enough, and if you have not been giving the body as many tools for the immune repair as for immune destruction, the body will not have what it needs to fully repair the damaged arterial walls. The lesions then remain partially unhealed, and plaque starts to build up in them.

Chronic Inflammatory Syndrome – seen in heart attack, stroke, and other vascular related diseases.

3 markers to watch especially for cardio- vascular disease, see previous page;
1. Fibrinogen – coagulation protein, high levels can induce a heart attack. Fibrinogen coagulates or thickens blood and includes increased platelet aggregation.
2. C-Reactive Protein – another inflammatory indicator, and indicates an increased risk for destabilized atherosclerotic plaque and abnormal arterial clotting.
3. Homocysteine – An indicator on how efficient your body (cells) repair and detox themselves.

Low fibrinogen, homocysteine or C-Reactive protein – you have a chance of living a relatively normal life.
Supplements that assist inflammation and vascular disease;
Nettle Leaf extract (most effective), and both Vitamin K and DHEA.
Supplements that assist in reduction and protection of <u>Fibrinogen levels</u>;
Vitamin C 2000mg per day, Niacin flush free 1000mg, EPA from fish oil 2800mg per day, bromelain 2000mg. Others include; vitamin E, low dose aspirin, garlic, ginkgo, and green tea extracts.
Hawthorn berry – improvement of blood supply to heart, dilation of coronary vessels.
Supplements that reduce <u>Homocysteine</u> levels;
Trimethylglyceine (TMG) 500mg, Folic acid 800mcg, B12 200mcg, choline 250mg, Inositol 250mg, Zinc 30, B6 100mg.

Heavy Metals (See also Toxins)
Chelated vitamins and minerals are the main ones to detoxify the body Fresh fruits also to assist detox and cleansing. Coriander has good benefits. Plenty fresh water to help flush system

High Blood Pressure
The heart pumps blood through the blood vessels, which can expand and constrict to suit. Note: The minerals Sodium/Potassium & Calcium/Magnesium need correct balance & this effects BP. Too

much salt constricts, Potassium relaxes the vessels. So, water, Potassium & Magnesium lower BP. See also pH of body in Addendum.

Remedy

FOODS required to reduce & maintain normal blood pressure; **Garlic & onions**, **nuts & seeds** [linseeds],or their oils (low H.I. factor), green leafy vegs. grains & legumes (fibre), Vitamin C foods esp. broccoli & citrus fruits. Other – **Hawthorn Berry**, take for 2 weeks for results) and has excellent cardiovascular effects – reduced deposition of cholesterol on artery walls, improvement of blood supply to the heart by dilation of coronary vessels, improves metabolic process of the heart thereby increasing force of contraction of heart muscle – results in lower BP. Contraindications / toxicity – very low
Iridology – <u>Faded iris colour</u> of the eye seen in high BP.
Systolic BP – highest pressure in blood vessel.
Diastolic BP – lowest pressure that remains in the artery when heart is at rest.
Symptoms of high BP (may not show symptoms at all)
Nosebleeds, dizziness, ringing in the ears, fainting spells, morning headaches, blurred vision, depression, urinating at night.
Normal range Blood Pressure
110/70 to 140/90

Pulse Pressure

Eg. 120/60 = 60 This is the pulse pressure and is the difference between Systolic and Diastolic readings of your blood pressure. Should be below 60, **30 – 40 is desirable (Check with your doctor)**

Foods to take

Vit C 500mg – 1000mg daily (+bioflavonoids)
Onions including garlic (all raw as possible). Linseed oil and fish oil Omega 3 and 6, and the pulse foods; beans, and peas.
Herbal – Hawthorn Berry extract, Black Cohosh

Also note; Calcium, B6, Potassium (help fluid balance), Magnesium (watch in kidney and heart disease), Coenzyme Q10,

Avocado – mild vasodilator that relaxes blood vessels and has a BP lowering effect.

Whole grains and legumes, (beans, lentils..) green leafy vegetables for their rich source of Calcium and Magnesium. Vitamin C rich foods such as broccoli and citrus fruits to help strengthen capillary walls and help clean blood vessels.

10 points to lowering high BP

1) Exercise – tones vessels, clears blood of excess fats and sugars, gardening is relaxing, 2) Run in place for six minutes, 3) Starting with leg muscles tense each group and hold for several seconds, 4) Take a long walk, concentrate on nature's beauties, sky colour, trees, etc. 5) Deep breathing – breathe with diaphragm. 6) Diet – Minimal stimulants (coffee, chocolate, spices, cheese [contains substance tyramine capable of constricting blood vessels and causing headaches]), Eat freely or fruits, vegetables, whole grains, SALT reduce antacids, baked goods, Fats remove of animal origin, 7) A vegetable diet for 3 days is good, apples are good to consume in fasting if need be, 8) Ensure body does not chill as this shunts blood from the extremities and taxes the nervous system, 9) Short hip bath – beneficial in lowering BP. Water at 18C for 3 minutes, reduce water temp, 10) Neutral bath – 10-30 mins neither warm nor cold, this calms the body. A hot bath at 40C for 20 mins will reduce BP. After bath cool gradually while lying in bed. After 30mins take regular shower.

Note: Check with your doctor before undertaking any changes or alterations to your health and lifestyle.

Human Intervention (Known as HI foods)

Any food that is altered, processed, etc, in some way is not optimum food for our bodies, and often our system cannot deal with it correctly, thus adding to more burden. It is important to pay attention to 'HI' foods and not so much on 'GI' foods. The more we process and intervene with foods, the more we consume altered foods that the body CANNOT process correctly. This taxes the body system, and adds to the toxic overload.

Illnesses

It is vital that you address your diet; preferably see a Naturopath/ Natural Therapist if illness persists.
Lazy organs, especially the digestive system and colon, allow rubbish to accumulate leading to health problems / illnesses. If you are constantly coming down with something and always fighting infections you really need to address your nutrition and lifestyle. You could also have poor nutrition that does not allow the immune system to do its' job. The immune system may be compromised and you will be aging the body faster than normal. Constantly ill, then also check protein intake. You must maintain certain amino acids from proteins to aid the liver to detoxify the body.
Remedy for colds - Garlic, Ginger, Fenugreek seeds combined. Boil and strain, add honey and lemon and sip regularly.

Wheat grass juice excellent all round cure if you have access to this product. To make this yourself place a thick layer of wheat seeds on a tray with soil. Once they're 8 - 10 cm. high, cut them with scissors, (they will keep growing), then vitamize shoots in a blender or juicer and drink the contents. Can be diluted. Try it! Also check for poor digestion – if your body does not digest foods correctly then you are not getting the benefit from the foods to help strengthen your body. This is also affecting your immune system.
Stubborn illnesses; a short fast required with one herb, for example; celery seed tea.

> **Most all illnesses are linked to nutritional deficiency patterns in some manner.**

We need some 70 + nutrients per day to stay healthy. Our bodies are resilient and can store some nutrients, however, most nutrients need topping up daily.

Inflammation

Inflammation is a sign of the body's reaction to some irritant, even though inflammation is a mechanism that is used in the body to overcome issues.
Inflammation can lead to excess mucous production as the body attempts to 'repair' the damage caused, and attempt to subdue the result.
An example would be:
Someone who is always having respiratory issues; always 'nasally' with blocked nose and clearing the throat. This mucous is as a result of an irritation, an inflammation effect from some issue.
Here, one should investigate what the *cause* of the inflammation is.
A test for levels of C-Reactive Protein, an inflammatory marker, will help with the indication of inflammation.
Inflammation can be useful as the body helps to repair a problem, but, can become chronic in which the inflammation causes further issues in your health maintenance.

Immune System

Regular sessions at the gym, (or other formats of weight resistant and aerobic exercise), will help keep your immune system efficient. A well-balanced diet with plenty of fresh fruit and vegetables and whole grains will provide most of the essential nutrients you need. Garlic and Ginger is excellent. Keep the bowels clear, so toxins aren't absorbed back into the body. Fresh fruit and vegetables as usual to keep the blood supply clean.

Sugar reduces immune system function

High fat diet suppresses immune system

Most people, especially kids, don't eat foods that contain Vitamin E.
Beta-carotene – the number of T-helper cells jumped 30% in study after men took 180mgs of beta-carotene a day for two weeks. (T-helper cells are important components of the immune system.)
Your immune system depends on; white blood cell function, genetics, environmental pollutants, our thoughts, emotions, stress levels,

personality styles, <u>foods we eat</u>, the digestive and absorption ability of our digestive system, toxins in our body and the foods we consume and some medications, to name a few.

Diet, supplements and lifestyle factors profoundly affect the health of the immune system.

Foremost amongst the micronutrients are the antioxidant vitamin and minerals, especially Vitamin C and E, beta-carotene, coenzyme Q10, Zinc, and Selenium. Thiamine (Vit B1), Pyridoxine (Vit B6) and Magnesium are also important. Garlic enhances the cytotoxic (cell killing), effects of phagocytes, and yoghurt (esp. cultures with L. bulgaricus), has wide ranging benefits. Yoghurt produces wide-ranging beneficial effects on the immune system. It greatly increases antibody and interferon production and causes increased production of natural killer cells. Fish oils also have a marked beneficial effect on many areas of the immune function.

Vitamin C benefits for the immune system

Vitamin C is the micronutrient most essential to the immune system. Leucocytes (white blood cells) cannot work without it. The body cannot store it, therefore, <u>we need to take in Vitamin C daily.</u>

Vitamin C and E inhibit the formation of two prostaglandins (PGE2 and PGF2), thus exerting an anti-inflammatory response and enhancing T cell production. (immune system)

A vigorous immune surveillance system is essential to help prevent the initial damage to a cell by a carcinogen and to allow the macrophages to destroy any metastasized cancer cells in the blood stream <u>before they can lodge in tissue.</u>

Antioxidants and immune deficiency

Deficiency in Selenium or Vitamin E – both antioxidants – can convert a latent, inactive virus into its active, disease causing form. This can explain why Selenium is effective against cold sores and shingles, which are both caused by reactivation of a dormant herpes virus. Maintaining correct immune system function and enhancing this through efficient antioxidant requirements, *greatly reduces the ageing effect on our bodies.*

What you eat can strongly influence the performance of white blood cells, the frontline warriors against infection and cancer. These are the neutrophils that engulf and kill bacteria and cancer cells, and the lymphocytes that include the T-cells, B-cells and natural killer (NK) cells. Yoghurt (L. Bulgaricus) has wide ranging benefits on the immune system. It increases antibody and interferon production and natural killer cells. Avocado – immune system stimulator and enhances antibody production. If you have low immunity then you may be more susceptible to infection, illnesses, cancer, etc.

Suggested dietary supplementation to enhance immune function

Vitamin C 1000mg, morning and night. Vitamin E 250mg per day (Do not take if on anticoagulant medication – consult with your doctor). Vitamin B1, 50mg in morning. Vitamin B6, 50mg in the morning. Beta-Carotene, 15mg per day. Coenzyme Q10, 30 to 60mg per day. Zinc 15mg per day. Selenium, 100micrograms (as Selenium) per day. Magnesium, 100mg (as Magnesium) per day. Evening primrose oil/fish oil 2 *1000mg capsules per day. Nutrient deficiency seen in diet therefore, weak immune system.

Foods to Eat

Green vegetables especially beneficial. An Italian study of breast cancer saw a one third reduction for women who consumed some green vegetables every day.

Grow your own vegetables. Not only will you save money the health of your family will benefit from these natural and wholesome foods.

Insomnia

Take;

Chamomile tea, Tryptophan foods (Walnuts, Chick Peas, Wheat Germ, Vitamin C, Turkey (the dark meat is better), Magnesium, Omega 3 oils. Address stress, at work and home, and look at other causes. Deep seated concern and worry – then find someone who can offer a solution to your dilemma, do not suffer it through as most times we can find solutions to problems by seeking others guidance.

Diet has a bearing on insomnia as well. Try limiting heavy meals to before six o'clock at night. The age-old saying works well; eat like a king at breakfast, eat like a queen at lunchtime, eat like a poor person at dinnertime. The secret is not to overload the digestive process late in the day. This can also be judged by the amount and vividness of dreams; if your dreams are, 'full on', then look more closely at your diet. A person, who sleeps poorly, wakes to go to the toilet several times a night, shows the nervous system has not yet slowed down. The nervous system is awake and waking the bladder to function.

Herbal remedy – Gotu Kola is of assistance to help sleep inducement.

Iron Booster

Iron requires Vitamin C to be absorbed efficiently. Pulverize all your green herbs in blender with lemon / pineapple juice - great iron boost! Herbs - rosehips, garlic, liquorice, red clover and sarsaparilla. These herbs can have a laxative effect on the bowel speeding up waste removal. Low fat meats are OK just do not overdo it with meat consumption. (Excess meat consumption can contribute to constipation – see section on bowels and Intestinal Transit Time.

Irritable Bowel Disease – and other inflammatory bowel diseases.
See bowel section.

Kidneys

(Hint - If urine is clear, then good fluid balance; Urine dark, then depleted fluid, excess Vitamin B, stress, or a disease pattern).

See also section on water.

The kidneys remove waste from the body. A chill to the kidneys slows down uric acid removal. If you are slow to get going in the morning, this may point to the kidneys / adrenal glands. Juniper berry tea is good to maintain fluid balance.

Remedy

Remove salt from your diet. Consuming cherries, blueberries, or cranberries and drinking celery seed tea daily can lower uric acid waste. Rolled oats, asparagus, dandelion and most salad vegetables are good. The source of uric acid is, generally, purine content foods; meat, yeast, fats and refined carbohydrates.

Drink sufficient clean water to help flush toxins from the body. Eliminate sugars from the diet, replace with honey. Chocolate can increase risk of kidney stones.
LAW OF SIGNATURES – Try Walnuts (like cures like). That is; Walnuts are similar to the shape of the Kidneys and have a benefit in supporting them.
Stress, fear and anxiety affect the kidneys. Take care of your kidneys as they 'support' the rest of the body - that which affects the body, affects the kidneys. To keep cellular fluid levels balanced take both sodium and potassium at correct levels.
Celery seed or cranberry juice is excellent. Celery high in sodium, Juniper berry tea high in potassium. Sodium increases cellular fluids and potassium reduces cellular fluids. Kidneys are affected by acid forming foods.

Some signs to watch
Hard pimples or dark dots in pouches below the eyes can show presence of kidney stones. Dark area below eyes can show; lack of sleep, exhausted kidneys, or low iron intake or absorption.

Kidney Stones

Hard pimples or dark dots in pouches below the eyes can show presence of kidney stones.
Chocolate can increase risk of kidney stones. Excess Calcium being leached out of the body, not necessarily from food intake. If you have Kidney stones your nutritional intake is out of balance. An acidic body needs neutralizing and Calcium generally is called on to do this – resulting in acidic bodies, loss of Calcium from the bones (Osteoporosis patterns), and Kidney stones.

Learning Difficulties

If the child is being criticized, condemned, unloved or not encouraged to name but a few, then this may show as the child with a learning difficulty. (Note: Seek professional advice to eliminate physical or physiological problems first).

Remedy

Support that child; treat this child with the opposite mentioned above. Also, remove refined sugar and sugar products from the diet <u>completely!</u>

Leg Cramps

Especially for those over 50 years of age can be a sign of inadequate digestion and poor assimilation of foods especially calcium, magnesium, potassium and other minerals. (See also section on diet.) Can also be a sign of a lack of Hydrochloric acid in the stomach.
Important – have your doctor check your heart and circulation, and check for atherosclerosis!

Liver (See also Gall Bladder)

(Hint - Unexpressed and suppressed emotions and anger are seen in the liver, so if you, 'fly off the handle' regularly, then signs are there that the liver may be stressed or dysfunctional.)
'The liver cleanses the blood; the more polluted the blood, the more the liver must work to eliminate the toxins. If these poisons stay in the liver, they affect the organs' health and efficiency.' Toxins not only include the obvious but also can include waste from daily cellular activity in the body.
Our modern day foods are truly not suited for the liver to deal with effectively. (See digestive system.)
A healthy liver is crucial to detoxify free radicals and toxic chemicals. (Make up, bathroom products, etc., contain toxic chemicals, also.)

Note: To deactivate chemicals in your blood, your liver needs helpers – nutrients such as B vitamins, minerals, omega-3 and amino acids to assist the detox process. If you are not getting enough of these key essential nutrients, your liver cannot work on its own – the liver will send chemicals back into the blood stream, without deactivating them. The need for detox is often seen where there are skin complaints and eruptions – psoriasis, eczema, ulcers, etc. You will need to see a qualified practitioner if you have ulcers and other blood borne disorders. Remember, the main function of the liver is to cleanse the blood of toxins and store the blood; take care of your liver watch the foods you consume!

Remedy

Foods that assist the liver to detoxify and function correctly are; **green** vegetables (especially cabbage, asparagus and sprouts), as raw as possible, avocadoes and walnuts. Onions are good also and consumed as raw as possible.
Herbs: Dandelion taken regularly is THE most effective herb to stimulate the liver. Swedish bitters is excellent also. Both products assist peristalsis of the digestive system helping the body to rid itself of toxins and wastes. Try it!
Lecithin, available from health shops, assists in cleansing the liver and breaking down cholesterol. Onions, again, are effective also. Vitamins A and D, plus a change to dandelion coffee, lemon grass tea and carrot juice for a period of time will tip the balance back towards optimum health.
Yoga style stretches and hot fomentation packs (over the liver), to improve circulation.
Nutrition includes; Selenium, omega-3, vitamin E and C, zinc, magnesium, vitamin B6 and glycine.
Liver detox include the above plus vitamin A/beta-carotene.

Cirrhosis – Chronic inflammation of liver cells leading to degeneration of healthy tissue. Inflammation produced by free radicals generated by viruses, toxins, bad fats, alcohol, drugs.
Increase antioxidants – VitC 1000mg 3 times a day (The most powerful

antioxidant for the liver)
VitE 1000iu+ (Natural VitE only eg. D-alpha tocopherol,) and Selenium 200mcg daily, (pref. 1-Seleniomethionine).

Early warning signs of Cirrhosis(possible) – Feeling tired, itchy, not sleeping, memory and focus problems and bouts of abdominal pain

Foods for the liver – Cruciferous vegs (broccoli, cauli, cabbage, kale, Brussels sprouts, bok choy, radish have indoles and sulphur for phase 1 and 2 detoxification process of the liver)

Cabbage is excellent contains **indole-3-carbinol** (I3C) and diindolylmethane and help to initiate liver detoxification. Indoles, found in cruciferous vegetables, are excellent support for women's hormones and general health – do not boil, light steaming or raw!

Turmeric and beetroot excellent for the liver.

Healthy Liver

A healthy liver is crucial to detoxify free radicals and toxic chemicals. (Make up, bath room products, etc., all contain toxic chemicals, as does some processed foods.

What you can do

Cruciferous vegetables – Brussel sprout, cauliflower and broccoli.

Cabbage is excellent it contains a crucial enzyme if you like called **indole-3-carbinol** (I3C) and diindolylmethane and helps to initiate liver detoxification. (Consume raw as possible).

Leukemia

Deficiency in **Folic acid** always seen. Folic acid needed for DNA and RNA. Dairy products may aggravate leukemia.

Longevity

Many groups of people around the world do not get our 'modern day' illnesses and diseases. Many live a very healthy life and over one hundred years in age. Groups such as; Abkhazians of Russia, Valcabambans of Ecuador and Hunzukuts of Pakistan are basically disease free. No cancer!

Reasons why;
They do not have processed foods, they consume around 70% high water content food – showing that natures' fruits and vegetables, seeds and grains are <u>what gives us life</u>. These natural foods contain 'all important' enzymes that nature provides.

Low Stomach acid / Malabsorption signs & remedies.

1. Eliminate known cause
2. HCl tablets trial to test for low acid production
3. Bitter foods to stimulate secretion; Dandelion, Sage, **Lemon Juice**, Garlic, Apple Cider vinegar, Swedish Bitters, Ginger, Licorice. Also take high dose Vitamin C powder for 2-4 weeks, then reduce for a period.
4. Digestive assisting enzymes; Bromelain (pineapples), yoghurt

Malabsorption Signs (these are some to watch)

- Fingernail strength test for nutritional deficiencies (cracked, peeling, week)
- Low energy
- Recurring illnesses & low immunity
- Arthritis type ailments – poor digestion & malabsorption of vits., mins & lack of enzymes.
- Leg Cramps (esp. over 50's) – showing poor assimilation of Ca, Mg, K & others
- Dilated blood vessels in cheeks
- Food Allergies
- Bloating, belching, flatulence
- Acne & other skin disorders
- Undigested food in stools
- Indigestion, diarrhea, constipation
- Headaches

Other foods to assist the digestion process; garlic, red onions, celery, radish, pumpkin, flaxseed oil (kind on digestive system), turmeric (anti-cancer properties & stimulates digestion), and the herbs milk thistle, wormwood.

Further explanations

Elevated Ph interferes with protein digestion – permitting bacterial overgrowth, resulting in toxification of the system.
Rheumatoid Arthritis & little or no gastric acid (hypochlorhydria), go hand in hand. RA – check bacterial overgrowth in gut. As we get older our stomach's produce less acid & pepsin – this inefficiency is often accompanied by gas. Can be a sign of 'Progressive Stomach Failure'.
Ulcers are caused by disruption in the protective barrier (mucous/bicarbonate) – Helicobacter Pylori bacteria most often causes this. Intragastric pH value of stomach is <4, <u>acid suppressing drugs drive pH >5, allowing bacteria to thrive.</u> Poor protein absorption can lead to food allergies. Antacid preparations reduce acidity & increase the risk of pathogens colonizing. Bacteria cannot survive in a highly acidic environment

YOU NEED A STRONG 'ACID BARRIER'

Lymphatic System

Lymph cleansing can best be achieved with iron, as this burns out the toxic rubbish from the system.
Ginger, lemon, garlic, onions (especially red onions), are good, along with herbs like nettle, red clover, gentian and rosehips.
Aromatherapy and massage - grape seed, grapefruit and juniper oils are good.
Avoid coffee and other mucous producing foods, as this only adds to an already overloaded lymph system. (See also acid producing foods). The lymph system has no pump to speak of to remove the waste, here exercise is extremely important. If lymph glands are enlarged then they are fighting something. Your lymph nodes are under the jaw, under the arms, back of the neck and above the groin. Seek professional advice.

A regular supply of <u>fresh fruit</u> & vegetables & freshly made juices are most beneficial for cleansing of the lymphatic system & therefore provide protection against the numerous infections & viruses that continue to develop in this modern society. When excess fats &

manufactured foods are ingested they can easily upset the functioning of the lymphatic system & illnesses, colds, viruses & poor health will likely be the prevailing result. Natural foods provide complete protection from infection.

The lymphatic glands are responsible for cleansing the body fluids, blood & by-products from digestion. The spleen is the largest organ within the lymphatic system & even though it is not essential to life, the spleen destroys worn out cells, red blood corpuscles & platelets.

Meal Preparation

(Hint: The more we cook, bake, or boil foods the less nutritional content these have).

When preparing meals for the family the aim is not to overcook or over heat foods, especially vegetables. The more we cook vegetables then the less nutritional content they will have: It is one thing to say you have vegetables regularly, but, do they have the nutrient content as nature intended for healing our bodies? Some people boil vegetables for twenty or more minutes when lightly steamed or raw is more beneficial for us. Live enzymes of nature's plant kingdom are destroyed when we cook them. This, in turn, means that we do not get the FULL benefit of that plant. If you feel you need to cook vegetables so they become more, 'palatable' for the family then try using herbs, spices, lemon juice and others that can help with the consumption of these foods close to their natural state.

Tips on maximizing the nutritional benefits of foods when cooking
- Use cooking oil sparingly during the process and add some quality oils at the completion of cooking.
- Add herbs, parsley etc. at the end of cooking for valuable enzymes and nutrient content.

Meat

Takes four hours to digest, and our digestive system is not designed for meat. Some is OK. Meat putrefies producing toxins and amines that accumulate in the liver, kidneys and large intestine destroying good bacteria. Excess meat consumption depletes key pancreatic enzymes. *These same enzymes are used by the body for certain processes in modern day disease patterns, also.*

Meat tends to encourage formation of inflammatory agents in the body. You will often notice big meat eaters that seem to have a 'nasally' voice when they talk. This can be a sign of excessive mucus in the body as a result of the inflammatory process when consuming incorrect or excess foods. Meat has no fibre to speak of and tends to slow down in the digestive tract: Big meat eaters will generally, have slow bowels, therefore absorbing more toxins into the blood stream. Meat is OK, just moderate amounts are better for you.

Menieres Disease

Salt – remove from diet, take multi vitamin tablet.
Supplementation to include;
Especially Calcium, Magnesium, Potassium (Contra-indications: Consult your doctor before supplementing Magnesium. Potassium if you have diabetes or kidney problems). Vitamin E inhibits blood platelet aggregation.

Inadequate diet, deficiency in B Vitamins, poor circulation. Niacin (B3) a vasodilator, gives effective assistance. Raw vegetables, beans, seeds, nuts, seaweed, fish, low fat yoghurt. Onions, garlic, chilli, lemons, lettuce, fish, no spreads on bread, (wholemeal of course).
AVOID – processed / refined foods, food additives, caffeine and soft drinks!
Exercise!
Reduce fat – inner ear is sensitive to high blood cholesterol levels.
Reduce sugar foods intake. This adds to an acidic body.

Menopause

The herb Black Cohosh is excellent. So too is Chrysanthemum. Sage is an excellent tonic for the nervous system. This assists in hormone rebalancing. Vitamin E and Calcium are essential as well.

Remedy

Consume more Magnesium rich foods, especially greens, and less processed foods in your nutrition plan. Vegetables help to fortify the body and lessen the effects of Menopause. You also need to reduce processed foods, fatty foods, sugary beverages and others. (See acid/alkaline section).
Hormone replacement Therapy (HRT). Take the natural progesterone, no imitations and no estrogen on its own. Long term you will need to address; lifestyle, exercise and <u>diet</u>.
Also, remove acid producing foods and replace with alkaline producing foods. (See acid / alkaline food section.)

Menstruation

(Hint - Question every product you take - as some pharmaceutical companies have a vested interest in the health industry.)

Amenorrhoea (lack of); try Chamomile and Potassium Phosphate.
Dysmenorrhoea (painful); improve nutrition and blood supply, see Liver section. Raspberry leaf tea is good.
Biochemical treatment; Magnesium Phosphate alternate with Ferrous Phosphate.

Period Pain - <u>then improve nutrition; exercise regularly, especially Yoga style stretches.</u>
Herb Cramp Bark is good for relieving pain. Chrysanthemum is good also.
Try this;
2 tablespoons of dried Cramp Bark and one tablespoon of fresh Ginger root in a pan with 3 cups of water. Add a cinnamon stick and a teaspoon of Fennel seeds. Cover and boil, and simmer for 10 minutes. Sweeten

with honey and drink it hot. This formula is anti-spasmodic and improves circulation, which is what you are trying to do.

Raw beetroot is excellent taken regularly. Carrot, beetroot and parsley combined in a blender are heaven for these patterns. Other herbs try Chamomile, Evening primrose oil or Valerian.

Minerals (see also: Vitamins)

Minerals are essential for many enzymatic and bodily functioning: They are the, 'switch' that turns on certain things in the body. Vitamins, on the other hand, build and support the functioning of the body.

For example; Iron, a well known metal element, is an essential component of blood. Zinc, another metal, supports the immune system. Selenium - true antioxidant and anti-cancer mineral.

Selenium is found in seafood and grains and seeds grown in soil containing Selenium. Check hydroponically grown produce for selenium content!

Mineral imbalances

Mineral imbalances can be linked with many autoimmune illnesses from Chronic Fatigue Syndrome, Coeliac Disease, allergies, Thyroid conditions, Arthritis and many others.

Remedy for deficiencies

Ensure a balanced diet that includes fresh fruits and vegetables, nuts and grains. See your health practitioner that is versed in nutrition and can help further with supplementation. However, do not rely on supplements alone.

Mucous (See dairy products and nutrition)

Mucous accumulation complicates the body's systems especially the inner ear, hay fever and hearing problems. Cysts, tumors and cancers are seen with mucous congestion as well.

- *You will also see excess mucous being produced by the body as a reaction to internal inflammation as the body tries to eliminate it. This reaction is likely from foods you are consuming.*

If you sound 'nasally' when speaking then there is probably a lot of mucous being produced and can be a sign of internal inflammation, and excess acid forming in the body. This is more than likely caused by incorrect nutrition! (See section on acid/alkaline balance.) Slippery Elm, found in good health shops, is mucilaginous – it will clear up mucous and pass it down through the intestines. Slippery Elm is a ground powder and is available at good health shops.

Nerve Conditions

Remedy

To overcome painful nerve conditions we need to cleanse and detoxify our bodies. Drinking lots of clean liquids is extremely helpful for neuropathy. Removing metals from the body is another important step. The body accumulates metals and the nerves in the lower extremities begin to degenerate as the levels in the body rise.

Remove metals in the body by undergoing chelation therapy. People find that pins and needles sensations and circulation improves. Vitamin C mega doses are excellent.

So Calcium, Glutathione, and other nutrients known to go into the cells to feed, nourish, and enhance the methylation and proper oxygen utilisation. Red juices are good – cherry, cranberry, raspberry and blueberry spiked with Vitamin C powder.

Night Blindness

Zinc is required for the enzyme that activates Vitamin A in the visual process. A deficiency of the enzyme can result in night blindness. Pumpkin and Sunflower seeds contain good zinc source, and leafy green and yellow vegetables and fruit for the Vitamin A and beta carotene content – <u>lightly steam vegetables</u>, **do not over cook!**

Obesity

Obesity is the 'result' of depression / stress. Can be a sign of boredom or minimal motivation in life.

Remedy

Seek out help! See a Counsellor or Psychologist that can help find the problem and assist you with a solution. Obesity is not so much heredity – it is inheriting bad diet advice.

Oedema (See Kidney section.)

Seen in an unbalanced diet and acid producing food intake – consult your practitioner.

Remedy

1. Eliminate salt from your diet!
2. Eliminate inflammatory producing foods and acid forming foods
3. Exercise and drink sufficient water, (no sweet drinks)

Can try Dandelion Tea.
Lymph drainage massage essential.
Aromatherapy - Juniper, Lemon, Rosemary, Grapefruit

Oils

Olive oil (extra virgin, cold pressed), Coconut oil (unprocessed is best) and linseed oils are good for us all. A note on oils: The coating of cells of the body need to be porous to allow good nutrients in and waste out of the cells. Heavy trans fats coat the cells with a hard layer reducing the transfer of nutrients. What an important consideration when you think of how our cells work at a minute level.

Margarine and other <u>hydrogenated</u> oils can be carcinogenic, therefore, they are not suitable to use.

There are margarines on the market that claim to reduce cholesterol – avoid them! These foods are acid forming in the body and do add to an already 'clogged' venous system in the body. It is the other 'products' that go into margarine and how it is processed that is not good for you. Natural foods such as Avocados and onions are excellent.

Pain Relief

For pain of joints and muscles try using powdered charcoal. Charcoal is soothing, antiseptic and <u>absorbs</u> vast amounts of toxins. Applied topically mixed to a paste. Try ice packs to remove heat and reduce inflammation. Cayenne Pepper is effective; boil in water, let cool and apply to area.
Wintergreen oil is good, massaged into the affected area as it contains salicylate – a similar constituent to aspirin, but is a natural way to reduce the pain. External use only!

Pantry

Your pantry needs to be part of your overall healthy lifestyle. Items to address include; replacing packaged cereals with whole rolled oats, sugar laden spreads out the door, even snacks such as potato crisps can be replaced with healthy alternatives. It's the little adjustments that make the difference. Use herbs and spices in your meal preparation regularly. Some that you can use include; turmeric, ginger, coriander, cumin, cinnamon and chilli powder. Shy away from salts and sugars as much as possible. Sugar is acidic for the body and salt retains fluid and excess fluid in the cells is not good for your health. Salt contributes to high blood pressure because of this extra fluid retention in the blood system. Honey, cold extracted of course, is the only choice as some honey brands are heat treated resulting in loss of nutrients. Pay attention to the stocking of your pantry. If you have snacks in the pantry then replace the commercial ones with healthy alternatives such as; wheat biscuits that have no fat added or salt.

Precautions in supplementation for health conditions.

Potassium supplements over 100mg NOT recommended.

Especially for; Diabetics, Kidney disease, NSAID,s takers, ACE Inhibitors, heart medicines such as heparin. Vitamin E – check with your GP if had previous stroke or blood problems.

Anticoagulant medication – if you prescribed this then should not take Vitamin E supplements.

Note: This is not a conclusive list check with your health practitioner.

Pregnancy and Supplements

Vitamin A in excess can cause deformities or death of foetus.
10,000 IU or lower are safe.

Potassium supplements over 100mg NOT recommended

NOTE: These are not the only precautions, check with a competent health practitioner.

Prostate *(See also section on glands)*

Remedy

Saw Palmetto (an age old useful herb)<u>is excellent</u>. Is a diuretic and urinary antiseptic and has a hormonal action to address the underlying problem.

Quit smoking, eat raw tomatoes and other raw vegetables especially those that are loaded with anti-oxidants.

Eliminate coffee, tea, alcohol and sugar. Address ongoing diet.

Also, take pumpkin seeds daily as these contain zinc, which is beneficial. Pumpkin and Sunflower seeds excellent for the Zinc content and essential fatty acids, which are essential for a healthy prostate.

<u>Pumpkin seeds</u> contain plant hormones that inhibit conversion of testosterone into the potent dihydrotetsosterone (DHT) form. <u>Tomatoes</u> contain the antioxidant lycopene, which is of great benefit in helping to prevent BPH and prostate cancer. Tomatoes are a good source of antioxidants.

Any drugs, (good or bad, antihistamines, etc.), can turn a partially obstructed prostate into a fully obstructed one.

Respiratory Complaints
Pneumonia

Vitamin A linked to decreased resistance to Pneumonia. Consume especially leafy green vegetables. Keep the immune system strong! You may need to see a qualified practitioner for some sound advice.

Rheumatism

The need is to <u>detoxify the system</u> - remove waste matter that congests and irritates muscles. (See a qualified natural practitioner, Naturopath, etc.) Digestive system attention is highly recommended, this will also assist with optimum absorption of nutrients. It is no good taking vitamins if the digestive system will not absorb them. Cleanse the system gently and replace with a good nutrition plan. (See Low acid diet plan.) The liver is quite often overloaded. Dandelion is excellent taken as a tea, or raw in a salad.

<u>Remedy</u>

Red clover to remove waste, dandelion, sage, ginger to improve circulation. Fresh fruit and vegetables (leafy green and iron rich), yoghurt and celery seed tea.

Please note; when eating vegetables eat them raw as possible, as cooking them depletes the natural enzymes and some vitamins and minerals that are required for a healthy body.

Eliminate instant coffee, processed foods and dairy products.

Food allergies; check for dairy, wheat, beef, tomatoes and peppers. A Fasting diet is good for Rheumatism.

70/30 Rule

Consume 70% natural foods containing 70% water content and 30% solid matter.

Why?

The earth is 70% water; we are 70% water so it is conducive to consume 70% water content foods for the correct functioning of the human body.

These foods are, generally, <u>most fruits and vegetables</u>. This is where true health starts. If you can maintain this ratio you will be a lot more healthier in the future.

Sickness

(Hint - The underlying cause to sickness is our own disorderly way of life!)

Sicknesses, physical and mental, never arise without cause, and the underlying cause, in all instances, is our own disorderly way of life.

Sinus

(Hint: Can be a sign of an irritated internal system that is acidic and producing excess mucous to compensate).

Avoid ALL dairy products; they are mucous producing for the body. Look strictly at your diet. Remove acid producing foods as these create a permanent state of panic in your mucous linings. Some common foods are; milk, processed cheese, sugar, meat, white bread, take-away foods, alcohol and cigarettes.

Remedy

<u>Treat the large intestine and eliminate constipation. Once stagnation is eliminated, sinuses open and lungs clear.</u> (See digestion section). Lecithin, Sulphur / Chlorine foods like cabbage and onions, parsnip, cucumber are good.

Help to get your body back to an alkaline base. (See section on acid/alkaline)

Skin Problems

If you have skin disorders, especially Psoriasis or Eczema, then you the problem may be internal. These problems are generally seen where there is poor elimination in the body and the body is toxic or acidic to a degree. This is a general comment and you would need further advice before acting on it.

Psoriasis

Caused by poor diet, poor digestion (especially of proteins) and build-up of toxins. Points to poor blood condition, and showing signs of excess heat within the body, according to Oriental diagnosis. The skin is indirectly linked with the large intestine, therefore, any health problems seen in the large intestine can manifest as reactions of the skin.
Faulty digestion is a known contributor. Toxic overload is found in patients with this disease.
STRESS – is known to be a great contributor.

Remedy

Linseed oil – reduces inflammation and kind on digestive system.
Fish oils may help to prevent and relieve the symptoms. The part of the fish most effective is eicosapentaenoic acid (EPA). Also cut back on pro-inflammatory animal fats and Omega-6 type vegetable oils, such as corn, sunflower, and safflower oils and <u>margarines and shortenings</u> made from them.

Other remedies
Herbs - red clover, dandelion, sage, liquorice, sarsaparilla and vervain help.
Also refer to the section on acid/alkaline balance for more ideas. Liver function must also be improved so try dandelion, carrot juice, lemon juice or a little cayenne pepper.
Linseed oil and fish oils increase the Omega 3 fatty acid levels and is a primary recommendation.

Eczema

Linked to the quality of the blood. There are toxins in the blood more likely caused by poor quality or incorrect foods and / or poor absorption through the digestive tract. Recommend you see a Naturopath or G.P. to confirm malabsorption of the digestive tract.

The elimination and circulation function is compromised due to toxins and excess fat, sugars, refined foods and additives.

<u>Remedy</u>

Eliminate allergens, milk, eggs, peanuts and limit animal products. Dandelion tea, improve bowel function (see bowel section), Vitamins A, E and Zinc.

Gingko Biloba and licorice (the herb), assist as well. (Contraindications – excess licorice can raise blood pressure.)

Skin infections and sores

Grated potatoes and/or onions are good for drawing out infections, sores, skin cancers. Apply to gauze and tape on. Leave for several hours at a time.

Tiny Capillaries on face – Petechial haemorrages.

Petechial haemorrhages (tiny, broken veins on the face and neck), take high dose Vitamin C and bioflavonoids, Vitamin K and Rutin for short term. Alter dose for future.

Leg Ulcers

Signs of; Poor circulation, Diabetes or a depressed immune system. *Please consult your health practitioner: If ulcers do not heal there could be an underlying problem that is contributing.*

Powdered milk thistle seeds can be used to treat leg ulcers and varicose veins. Aloe Vera (fresh leaves) has good effect on leg ulcers and some other skin complaints.

Blisters, Wounds, Warts and Dry Skin *on the legs or feet is often due to imbalances in our biochemistry.* <u>***The more toxic we are, the more bacteria and viruses we have!***</u>

Diet for skin conditions

Start by eliminating all major allergens especially; milk (& dairy products), eggs, peanuts, and wheat can be a problem also. LIMIT animal products, fats etc. Include 'fatty' fish such as salmon, herring or mackerel in the diet. (These are the good fats contained in the fish.)

Supplements

Linseed oil (available from good health shops in the fridge section), or can use evening primrose oil. Linseed (Flaxseed) oil can go rancid easily and needs to be fresh and preferably not in capsule form.

FOODS to assist the skin;

Carrots, lettuce, beans, cucumber, currants, berries, dates, figs, cabbage. Carrots support the liver, lettuce cleanses along with cucumber and cabbage. Please consume these foods as **RAW** as possible. The more vegetables are cooked, the less plant hormones, enzymes and other essential elements are available for the body to use correctly. Nature provides these foods with the correct quantities and balance of nutrients.

Use the foods daily – proportionally more than any other foods.

Topical

Aloe Vera is unsurpassed as to the benefits it instils on the patient. Fresh leaf from a plant is best. Honey has good healing properties as well. Onions can be used for infections to draw out bacteria, etc. Bandage on a thick slice, (or half a small onion), over the infected area, and replace daily. Try it! You will be surprised at the properties of onions.

Internal

Licorice can be used safely and has great benefits – anti-inflammatory and anti-allergic effects.

Vitamin Mineral supplementation for skin

Eczema sufferers seem to lack certain vitamins and MINERALS. Take a quality multi vit/min tablet to ensure you are receiving sufficient nutrients. Plenty of fluids, and sufficient alkaline foods. Alkaline foods are, generally, fresh fruit and vegetables – not processed, packaged foods.

Spleen

(Hint: this is the organ of emotions and if emotions are not dealt with can overflow to the Liver.)

Low spleen function can lower your immunity, resulting in anaemic patterns of pale skin, weakness, loss of drive. Glandular fever and Leukaemia can then be possible.

Remedy

Beetroot taken raw (Doctrine of Signatures ie; like cures like). Sesame, Olive, grapeseed, corn oils are good. Avoid Canola, Sunflower and margarines as much as possible as these are hydrogenated and can be carcinogenic.

Sprays and chemicals on food crops

I have included this here because of its importance and relevance in our health. Nowadays some commercial crops, in the pre-harvest phase, have been sprayed with some chemical. Potatoes often have a weed killer sprayed on the tops to kill them off quickly so the farmer can get them to the supermarket on time. Onions can have the same spray used as well. Imported garlic and others often is fumigated to kill off bugs and yet this spray can be potent for us consumers.

If you think about it for a moment when you spray a potato plant, for example, the poor potato will absorb some portion of spray. This chemical we then ingest along with possible many others, and we wonder why we are getting ill!

To give you an example; many years ago, whilst my father was running the family orchard, and as part of the pest management program he used a spray regularly on apples to stop certain diseases and bugs. Many years later he was diagnosed with lead poisoning and this would undoubtedly have come from the chemicals used in the spraying process – just be aware!

What to do.

Source your vegetables and fruit from farmer's markets or other reputable natural sources as possible. Ask questions if it is possible about the origin and sprays used. Also, cut out the eyes of potatoes as this is where chemicals could concentrate. Rinse your vegetables well before use especially; broccoli, celery, potatoes and grapes. Even washed potatoes you buy can be washed with anything from straight water to strong detergents <u>and others</u>.

Stomach Ulcers

Most stomach ulcers are caused by a disruption in the protective barrier, (mucous / bi-carbonate), frequently caused by Helicobacter Pylori bacteria or aspirin or other non steroidal anti-inflammatory drugs (NSAIDS). A balanced diet is also required; and do not take antacid preparations. Please see your health professional for complete analysis.

Stomach Acid

Stomach acid kills bacteria! As we get older our stomachs don't produce as much acid and pepsin. Food is often accompanied by gas. We need a strong acid barrier to correctly digest foods, otherwise we see digestive complaints more often. Acid suppressing drugs drive stomach pH higher than 5, allowing bacteria to thrive. Low stomach acid conditions greatly contribute to nutritional deficiencies, even if you eat correctly!

Pepsin, required for the digestion process, cannot be formed at pH5 or higher. Protein digestion requires a low pH in the stomach, ie; good stomach acid production! What to do for low stomach acid conditions;

1. Eliminate cause
2. Bitters to stimulate
3. Lemon juice in water, Ginger or apple cider vinegar
4. Hydrochloric acid and pepsin supplementation taken with meals
5. Test stomach acid level (can use hair analysis for iron, calcium and zinc levels)
6. If chronic seek specialist advice

Stress

Stress – perceived inability to cope, based on what is going on in our heads versus the REAL outside world. Stress triggers major health problems and we age quicker. B group vitamins are also drawn on in times of stress. Learn how to switch off, support each other in times of stress. Talk with a counsellor as they can help with ideas and suggestions. Vitamin C powder supplementation is effective.

10 TIPS TO BEAT STRESS

1. Talk out your problem with a partner or close friend – this can be the best method,
2. Breathe – the more oxygen in your lungs the better our physical condition, and the clearer we think.
3. Exercise – proven beyond doubt, get out there, climb that mountain, have fun, you are entitled to it.
4. Meditate – excellent stress reliever best to work with a group to start off with and learn techniques.
5. Say 'No' - Every time you do something you don't want to a little stress builds up, learn to say no and people will respect you for it.
6. Get Creative – Break the monotony of your daily routine; take up a hobby, painting, music, etc., and other left brain activities will help to open up this creative aspect of you!
7. Make some 'Me Time' – goes without saying, just do it!
8. Get back to nature – this is overlooked and nature is so beneficial. Get your friends together and take a walk in nature.
9. Stop working – Learn to have balance in your life. Remember the old saying, "All work and no play makes Jack a dull boy"
10. Get organised – When life seems out of control, stress is inevitable. Get your daily planner out and write down your, 'to do' list. It does make a difference with your stress levels.

One final point;
EMOTION IS YOUR ENEMY,
TALENT IS YOUR GUARDIAN…
(Work with your talents and this will help to balance your emotions)

Sugar

Leaches the body of precious minerals and vitamins and produces an over-acid condition in the body, leaving the way open for diseases even cancers to take hold.

Supplements

Hint: Source reputable supplements from your health shop.

Vitamin and mineral supplements can be of assistance to your diet, but be aware of imitations. Supplements need to be formulated and synergistically balanced in their manufacture. They have to have the right amounts of vitamins and minerals in the right balance – just as nature has done in the foods we eat. Don't just pick up vitamin tablets from the local bulk store, etc. Talk with a qualified professional about the supplements you take.

Some supplements can go rancid quickly; fish oil is one of them! Try to vary the supplements you take. For example; you might take one supplement for a week, then change to another for a short period of time, then have a break for a week or two, etc. Remember, you get what you pay for and quality supplements need to be found.

Teeth

(Hint - brush twice daily, with quality toothpaste and floss regularly. Avoid mercury containing fillings.)

Use a stiff toothbrush to brush your teeth; the idea is to remove any plaque.

Calcium is needed in the natural form, not fluoride. Eliminate fluoride containing toothpaste!

Teeth decay seen in poor diet conditions, lack of key nutrients in the foods, a lack of calcium in the diet and excess sugars. The correct calcium is found in fruits and vegetables such as; cabbage, honey, sprouts, parsley, sesame seeds, spinach, kale, vegetable salt, kelp, almonds, bran, Brussels sprouts, broccoli, chick peas.

Fluoride causes bones to deteriorate; the thyroid to become underactive! Flouride does not support your teeth – according to the latest research, Calcium does! Sodium Lauryl Sulphate (SLS) used in some commercial toothpastes, is a poison. Often listed on toothpaste with, ' derived from coconuts.' Yes, but is prepared with sulphur trioxide or other chemicals. Avoid it!

Tooth fillings - request 'non - mercury' containing fillings. Source a reputable calcium-based toothpaste without SLS or fluoride additives.

Reason: Your teeth have tiny tubules and can absorb minerals – hence calcium absorption. My wife and I use a high calcium content toothpaste derived from coral and have great results.

Loose teeth can be a sign of poor nutrition. Check with your dentist, (or Naturopath), for more information. If you have to use tooth paste, *use it sparingly*!

Tests

(Hint – ask your doctor to check your Homocysteine, C-Reactive Protein and Fibrinogen blood levels in your blood, especially if you are over 50 years of age. See Heart section.)

Three tests you should have done regularly through your doctor;
1. Homocysteine – high levels shows pre-disposition to atherosclerosis and heart attack, and is a good indicator of <u>reaction to inflammation in the body</u>.
2. C-Reactive Protein – indicates inflammation processes and is also linked to heart and vascular problems,
3. Fibrinogen – is a clotting factor produced in the liver, and excess fibrinogen can indicate cardiovascular disease.

Other tests you can do at home (for information purposes only, <u>do not self diagnose</u>)
- Fingernail
    Fingernails that crack, peel or break easily can show nutritional deficiencies and/or lack of minerals. Can also show poor digestion in the stomach.
    Dents or ridges running across the nail can indicate infection or a disease or major stress
    Dents or ridges running the length of the nail can show poor health, possible kidney or liver disorders.
- pH of body fluids.
    You can test your urine or saliva pH using litmus paper available from pharmacies or good health shops. This can give you a

good indication how your body is performing inside. If acidic then adjust with your nutrition and diet plan. Recommend you do see a qualified health practitioner in this field for further advice.

- Allergy pulse rate test.

  Master this and you can tell which foods are suitable and which are not for your body.

  How to perform this simple test: Take your resting pulse reading: Consume a food item, wait approximately ten to fifteen minutes and check your resting pulse rate again. If there is a noticeable increase then the food is not conducive for your body. Once you master this you will be able to eliminate or include certain foods that benefit your health.

- Low stomach acid indicator

  If you suffer from heartburn take a tablespoon of apple cider vinegar. If this clears the heartburn in approximately twenty minutes then you may have low stomach acid. (Refer to section on digestion.) Note: If symptoms persist see your health professional.

Do not forget the usual checks of all important; blood pressure, cholesterol levels and others as prescribed by your doctor. What do these tests show you? <u>They can pre-warn you of probable future problems with your health</u> – **your early warning system!** Ask your doctor about these and other tests to perform.

Tolerance

I have included this here because we tend to be over-tolerant with matters of health, and life! If you tolerate something you will develop stubbiness to change be it; ill health situation, aches and pains or your work/career life. Try and develop the understanding that tolerance can have good and bad points: You may tolerate that pain in the chest. You may tolerate that job when you could take the leap of faith and look at other opportunities. Do not tolerate health concerns – you may need a second opinion from a qualified health professional and this could save your life.

Tongue

Your tongue can indicate your general health, especially the condition of the foods we eat.

Any fur coating, as it is known, on the surface of the tongue or unusual colouring is an indication of the wrong foods we are consuming and / or health problems. The tongue surface should be clear and clean as this indicates good digestion and circulation

Colour of the coating on the tongue

White coating indicates; excessive amounts of fat, dairy products, baked foods as these create congestion in the system. Can also be a sign of overeating. Black coating indicates; kidney problem and needs further exploration with a health practitioner. If you discover these colours consider a revamp of your nutritional and lifestyle plan. Check with someone qualified in natural health to determine the condition properly.

Toxins

Note: Toxic overload of our soils with modern fertilisers that contain heavy metals and extreme levels of Phosphorus are detrimental to our health.

These high levels are seen with our modern day illnesses.

To remove toxins you need foods rich in Calcium, Iron, Potassium, Magnesium.

AND important alkali ions of the Sulphate group:
Magnesium Sulphate (Epsom Salts), Potassium & Iron Sulphate. These help clean out toxins & greatly reduce acidity problems (modern day illnesses) and keep bad bacteria under control.
Cruciferous vegetables are excellent also.

Ulcers (see leg ulcers in Skin section)

Varicose Veins

Years of dietary mismanagement contribute to varicose veins. It is a little like the course of a river, where every bend is clogged and slowed down by a buildup of silt.

Description – The return venous system is compromised and valves in veins not efficient as should be.

Remedy

Lecithin, Vitamin E and C and exercise to start undoing years of dietary mismanagement.

Linseed oil, preferably under four months old, taken daily. Two tablespoons each day will help.

Garlic and onions (raw) are excellent! Sitz baths are good to improve circulation of the limbs. Sitz baths are taken first hot, then cold, then hot, then cold alternating for twenty minutes a day.

Bioflavonoids especially beneficial. Sources – blue berries, black berries, raspberries, kiwi fruit, rosehips, chillies and other citrus fruits and vegetables. Bioflavonoids strengthen capillary walls, and form collagen in connective tissue. Bioflavonoids assist Vitamin C in absorption. Rutin containing foods assist and these include cherries, rose hips and citrus fruits. Avoid junk foods, salt and refined and reduce processed foods. Keep your blood thin. (See section on blood).

Herbal – Gotu Kola Excellent! (enhances blood flow, increase tone of connective tissue. Bilberry compliments Gotu Kola.) Horse Chestnut helps control inflammation, swelling and <u>reduce</u> fluid accumulation. Eliminate hard SALTS!

Vitamin E – helps keep platelets, blood components involved in clotting, from sticking together AND adhering to the sides of the blood vessel walls. Dosage – 200 to 600 IUs daily is enough to assist in reducing platelet adhesion.

Contra-indications – consult doctor if you have had a stroke, bleeding problems, or use anticoagulants if you are going to take Vitamin E.

Red or blue spider veins – appear when fragile capillaries distend or break down. (A sign of lack of Vitamin C and bioflavonoids.) Lecithin, Vitamin E and exercise to start the repair.

Vegetables

(Hint – consume as raw as possible to receive optimum nutritional and enzyme content)

Grow your own!
One of the most important things you can do is grow some vegetables yourself. You may not be an avid gardener so here are some suggestions for you;

- Parsley and other herbs, in a pot near the kitchen. Remember the live enzymes in these foods.
- Border a small area, fill it with soil and fertilizer and plant common, hardy vegetables such as carrots, beetroot, silver beet, tomatoes, etc. Carrots and beetroot can last for months.

The plant kingdom is what helps to heal our bodies amongst many benefits. Using as many colored vegetables is recommended. Cruciferous vegetables are extremely beneficial – broccoli, cabbage, cauliflower, Brussels sprouts.
Some worthy facts about vegetables;

- Pulses- help lower blood cholesterol, stabilize blood sugar levels and are a good source of protein, minerals and Vitamin B
- Cruciferous vegetables (mentioned above), contain sulphureous compounds that help protect against some forms of cancer. Cruciferous vegetables also contain Indoles which is a Nitrogen compound that help speed up elimination of estrogen hormones from the body which may help to protect women from cancers.
- Green vegetables are loaded with plant chlorophyll. This compound found only in plants is nearly exactly the same as a molecule of iron in our blood. I have mentioned this point because one can see that consuming plants is conducive with our own chemistry – our own blood!

How to prepare vegetables for a meal
Do not boil or roast vegetables too much as key nutrients and enzymes are destroyed in the process. You need to consume vegetables

as raw as possible – light steaming is acceptable as this process retains nutrient content <u>and enzymes.</u>
Something to keep in, mind with fruits and vegetables;
> If the soil that the plant is growing in is devoid of certain nutrients, for example the mineral Selenium, then the plant will be deficient of Selenium. This is one main reason why we need to consider organic grown foods or those grown as naturally as is possible.

In fact fruits and vegetables have antioxidants in abundance to fight free radicals, which are a key cause of ageing.

Vitamins (and Minerals)

Ensure good intake of Vitamins and minerals in their NATURAL state. Consume foods that are rich in them and consume fruit and vegetables as raw as possible.

Vitamin C, E, A are all essential anti-oxidant vitamins, among others, that should be included in your diet – daily!

We need some 70+ vitamins and minerals daily to keep our body functioning correctly. Over time a deficiency of these can take a toll on our health – not so noticeable straight away but can make a HUGE difference in the future. Many illnesses and diseases are due to this long term deficiency; Arthritis, heart problems, the list goes on.

Vitamins and minerals summarized below. There are two groups of vitamins:

Water soluble – B and C vitamins. Absorbed rapidly and need to be taken in regularly (hence; this is why you need to take in health giving foods)

Fat soluble – vitamins A, D, E and K. These tend to be stored in the body for future needs.

Vitamin A

Excellent antioxidant; involved with RNA (cell coding), immune system, antibody production…

Sources; fish liver oils and salmon, cod etc.

Health indication; skin conditions like eczema, psoriasis, cancer prevention, asthma, allergies, Crohn's disease.

Toxicity: could be toxic above 25,000 I.U.

Vitamin B group

B1

Needs Folic acid for absorption. Functions include; essential for energy production, cofactor for more than 24 enzymes, involved in neuro-transmission.
Deficiencies include; heart problems, diabetes, burning feet…
Sources; Peas, lentils, brown rice, nuts, bread, beef, sunflower seeds.

B2, Riboflavin

Functions include metabolism of carbohydrate, protein and fat, maintains mucosal tissue, assists B6, aids red blood cell production.
Deficiencies include; Crohn's disease, blurred vision and cataracts, cracked lips.
Sources; Almonds, green leafy vegetables, eggs, avocados and meats.

B3, Niacin

Involved in energy production, excellent for lowering cholesterol, triggers bile and stomach secretions, hormone synthesis.
Deficiencies: pellagra (Dermatitis, Diarrhea and Dementia.
Sources; Meat, egg, almonds, legumes, sunflower seeds, whole grains and yeast.

B5, Pantothenic Acid

The 'anti-stress' vitamin. Involved in energy production, neurotransmitters. Treatment for; stress and depression, skin and hair, wound healing, eczema, asthma, arthritis.
Sources; Avocado, whole grains, oranges, beans, fish.

B6, Pyridoxine

This is a super nutrient involved in 60 enzyme reactions. (B6, B12 and Folic acid lower homocysteine levels in the body. Homocysteine is an inflammatory marker and is an indicator of internal inflammation in the body. (See section on inflammation).

Functions include; reduces risk of CHD, asthma conditions, kidney stones and lowers urea and blood oxalate levels, Coeliac disease, Parkinson's disease, depression, diabetes and osteoporosis.

Sources; Cauliflower, nuts, avocados, seeds, potatoes, egg yolk, fish and meats.

B12, Cyanocobalamin

Stored in the liver.

It plays a major role in manufacturing RNA (ribonucleic acid), helps maturation of red blood cells, involved in conversion of homocysteine to methionine and formation of healthy cells and myelin sheath of the nerves.

Deficiencies include; Pernicious Anaemia, depression, asthma, M.S., Crohn's disease.

Sources; animal foods such as meats, egg yolk. Vegetarians are usually deficient in B12.

Folic acid, Folacin, Folate.

Folic acid is an inseparable part of B group.

Functions include; RNA and DNA synthesis, prevention of spina bifida in newborns, reduces the risk of CHD (coronary heart disease), skin disorders like acne, psoriasis and prevention of cancers.

Sources; lentils, whole grains, cereals, broccoli, beans, oranges, peas, cabbage, eggs and liver.

Vitamin C

Strong antioxidant and protects many essential nutrients from oxidation. Helps remove toxins from the body. Deficiency of Vitamin C can be seen as easy bruising. Vitamin C combined with E will help combat inflammation in the body, (which may go on to cause other health problems; Arthritis, etc.)

Protects against diabetes and cancer.

Vitamin C should be taken in the most natural form if you are supplementing. The powder form is preferred over the coloured tablets you can purchase and these are not as effective or absorbed by the body correctly. Take bioflavonoids with Vitamin C to aid absorption. Bioflavonoids are antioxidant plant pigments that protect us from free radical damage. Citrus fruits are the main source and have <u>10 times the concentration in the pith and membranes.</u>

RDA (recommended daily allowance) was set many decades ago. The requirements of the human body have changed and need to consider higher doses. EDR (Effective Daily Requirement) is now more acceptable.

Note: Please do not rely on taking massive amounts of vitamin tablets. Remember, natural foods in their raw state are more beneficial. However, large doses of, for example, Vitamin C can be very beneficial to help some health
concerns. (See a health professional before making changes to the recommended dosage.)

This is not a conclusive description of vitamins although this offers some insight into the *importance* of a balanced intake of these and other nutrients – we need some 70+ nutrients daily just to maintain the health and functioning of the body.

Bioflavonoids

Bioflavonoids are antioxidant pigments from plants and fruits that protect us from free radical damage.

Rutin – is a bioflavonoid found concentrated in the pith of citrus fruits, the white core of green peppers, prunes, rose hips, apricots, cherries, rhubarb, mint, buckwheat and chamomile.

Benefits include; free radical scavenger, improves circulation, high cholesterol,, cirrhosis, cataracts, stress, hemorrhoids and constipation.

Main benefit –Strengthens capillary walls and regulates their permeability. This promotes capillary health. (Capillaries are the tiny blood vessels throughout the body).

Deficiency: Similar to Vitamin C deficiency and shows as <u>easy bruising</u>. Older people tend to bruise easy and this is accountable for this deficiency generally. Take note of this for the future.

> Minerals are essential in any nutritional plan because they are the switch, if you like, that have a huge impact on the correct functioning of other processes in the body.

Calcium

Calcium is essential for our bones, nerves and heart. It is a most abundant mineral and is the main one in the bones of the body. What is interesting is that if our bodies are acidic to some degree then Calcium is released from the bone structure to help neutralize the acid. What tends to happen is the body becomes deficient in Calcium and Osteoarthritis signs may start to show. The best source of Calcium is from vegetables and fruit. The reason is because Calcium from vegetables is more readily utilized than that found in dairy products. Dairy Calcium seems to be a hard Calcium that the body finds harder to assimilate or use it correctly. Sources of Calcium; green vegetables, broccoli, cabbage, silver beet, oranges and other citrus and is also in seafood, almonds, figs, prunes, tofu and sesame seeds. A little dairy is OK but keep this in check as mentioned, you get better availability of Calcium from the plant kingdom.

Magnesium

Magnesium and Calcium work together. It is utilized by numerous enzymes. As Magnesium is part of the chlorophyll molecule; fruits vegetables and grains are high in Magnesium. A very essential mineral indeed.

Zinc

Zinc is involved in many enzyme processes and this includes DNA and RNA production, (the genetic structure of ourselves if you like). Zinc is used by the body in functioning of the eyes, smell, taste, mental function and brain development. We cannot overlook the benefits for the immune system.

Iron

Iron is an essential mineral and is the most abundant trace element in the body, especially the blood system. It is vital for growth, the nervous system and immune system to name a few.
(There are other minerals that the body requires and you can see the importance of complete nutrition.)

Selenium

An essential trace element that is soil dependent. (If Selenium is not in the soil that the plant grows in then there will be none of this in the food it produces.) Selenium is involved in an extremely important antioxidant system within the cells. Selenium protects the cell membranes by helping prevent lipid peroxidation. (Cells of the body all have a delicate membrane that helps regulate the cell, letting in good nutrients and releasing the waste products of cell metabolism).
This is not a conclusive list just an indication of some of the main ones.

Water

(Hint – water maintains fluids for the body and helps to flush toxins out!)
Drink sufficient water for your circumstances, this will depend on your lifestyle, work and seasons of the year, among other factors. Do not over drink fluids excessively though.
You do not have to drink two litres of water a day as many diet recommendations suggest. Those of you with an unbalanced diet and excess toxins or a demanding job or exercise routine, will need to drink around two litres of water a day to assist the flushing action performed by the kidneys of the blood. Everyone has different requirements and, therefore, one rule does not fit all. Cool water is best, as the body does not have to work to bring the internal temperature back to homeostasis, your normal working temperature. Excess water can have an effect on the electrolyte imbalance.

If you need to drink during meals then the body is telling you it is lacking water during the day. Also, drinking during meals *disrupts the digestive process* – ideally you should not drink for an hour after a meal. Try having your drink before your meal. Drinking water keeps the kidneys flushed and toxins excreted via the urine. Enjoy!

Weight Loss
(Hint – Natural foods that nature produces is the way to better health!)
Remedy

Three important steps to permanent weight loss;
1. **'Paint the Picture'** results in advance. 'See yourself in the future, how you will feel, the compliments you will get, how healthy you will be, etc.

2. **Diets do not work!** Dieting starves the body of key nutrients and when you stop dieting the weight goes back on as the body is trying to tell you that it needs nutrition – not a large pie, cream cake, chocolate, etc.

3. **Take Action and Personal Responsibility!** Genetics does not have a lot to do with weight gain, as does a poor attitude and laziness. Have a simple healthy lifestyle plan that INSPIRES you to be healthy!

See your local fitness centre, Naturopath, weight loss centre and others that can help guide you correctly. Set a plan that is ACHIEVABLE! Train with friends Have steps set along the way Join a gym if you have trouble with motivating yourself – remember you are not alone!

<u>If you can't see yourself the new you in 12 months time – you won't commit!</u>
Simple exercise routine daily
- Standing squats, bend knees squat to near 90 degrees and hold for count of 3
- Push ups – bent knees or straight legs if you can. All the way down, watch technique.

- Isotonic stomach strengthening, with elbow and forearm on floor – hold for count of 5-10
- Dips on chair (triceps), do these strict and stretch as low as you can.

Do circuit 2-3 times and should take around 10-12 minutes. Maintain a strict form, going the whole range and holding for a count. This may seem a little harder at first, but you will see results sooner – you will only cheat yourself if you are not completing the whole routine correctly. Have some music that harmonizes you and makes you feel good. Enjoy!

Turn
FATS – Fear, Anger, Tension, Stress
   Into
FATS – Faith, Accept, Trust, oneself

Excess insulin suppresses the release of growth hormone, in addition to preventing fat from being released from cells in people trying to reduce body fat.
When the blood is saturated with insulin, the body will not release significant fat stores, even if you restrict your calorie intake and do exercise.

Worms (Intestinal and other parasites)

Worms and parasites thrive in an acidic environment. So, if worms return then your internal body may be over acidic thus supporting their cycle. Parasitic infections, if left untreated, weaken your body's defense system (immunity) because of blood loss, malnutrition and tissue damage. Other symptoms include; fatigue, nausea, abdominal pains and loss of appetite.

Remedy

Pumpkin seed kernels, pepitas, are unsurpassed in helping rid the body of parasites especially the intestines. Chick peas are a good cure for intestinal worms. Walnuts can help also.

Foods to consume include; garlic, raw onions, cinnamon, cloves, radishes and mustard.

Herbs to consume include; basil, allspice, curcumin, coriander, sage, rosemary and thyme have the best results.

Include the recommendations above in your daily nutrition plan for several days.

Worry

I have included this point in the health section as it **so** relates to health we cannot overlook the consequences of this.

Worry is a most highly destructive pastime, especially negative worry, when charged with emotion can bring about health problems. If you still can't see a link between worry and the mind, and our health then ponder the following point;

> In the sixteenth century the Swiss alchemist Paracelsus discovered that emotional thought patterns have long-term reactions. This discovery has since been confirmed by modern day psychoanalysts, who often locate the cause of a sleep disorder deep within the subconscious, born of the <u>fears</u> initiated during an earlier life experience.

Ways to deal with worry;

- In a journal write down the 'pros and cons' of the problem
- Meditate
- Walk in the park, bush, fresh air
- Talk with someone you can trust with matters of the soul, (that can be a tough one!)

Look at many options as you can to overcome your concern..

Low Acid Diet plan

Suggestions for meal replacement

For lowering acid in body and weight rebalancing.

Lemon juice 10 minutes before meal.

BREAKFAST – Rolled Oats not one minute oats, no sugar or dairy milk, sprinkle of nuts, almonds, etc. (No peanuts), dried fruit excellent. Fresh fruit, glass of veg./fruit juice (not commercial juice), toast (wholemeal only). Packaged cereals have minimal nutritional content or enzymes and can be acid forming in the body.

LUNCH – Boiled baby potatoes (no butter or margarine), served with diced tomato, capsicum, greens, herbs, etc., parsley, garlic. Glass of soy milk or herbal tea.

DINNER – Grilled fish (in extra virgin olive oil only), lightly steamed vegetables, banana, nuts, grains, yoghurt, herbal tea.

Other main meal substitutes; potatoes, rice, lentils, some pasta.

SNACKS (mid morning and afternoon) – berries, nuts, fruit, dried fruit, yoghurt. Try yoghurt and almonds, or, berries and dried fruit.

NO ADDED SALT – Affects the kidneys and heart directly.

On weekends when you have more time try preparing a more nutritious breakfast. For example; sliced tomatoes on toast, no margarine, an egg or two and some herbs to garnish – your body will thank you!

Most weekends for breakfast I have; steamed potatoes, silverbeet, an egg (free range), herbs, turmeric and lemon juice. (All alkalizing for the system.)

Healthy snacks to take to work try; grated raw beetroot, grated carrot, parsley or chives and lots of lemon juice. Take this in a small sealed container and enjoy! Your body will thank you!

If constipated then consume more fruit; pears, dates, apples, prunes, celery, lemons and bitter foods like dandelion that will stimulate digestion and peristaltic actions in the intestines. Linseed oil is very beneficial also, (a tablespoon of young oil).

Keep in mind;
> Too many sweet foods affect the spleen and are acid producing. Dairy products are in the same category of producing acid waste in the body and especially, settle in the joints. These can be often recognizable as aching stiff joints with limited movement, accompanied with pain, however, this is not the only cause of stiff joints.
>
> Too many purine foods (heavy red meats and organ meats) can produce more uric acid and contribute to further addition of wastes settling in the joints.

ALTERNATIVE FOODS

Ginger, garlic, onions, potatoes, green vegetables, berries, nuts (not peanuts), lemons, fruit, cabbage etc., tahini, soy products, sunflower seeds (contain antioxidant Selenium), pumpkin seeds (contain Zinc for the protection of the liver), olives, olive / linseed / grape seed / sesame / corn oils. Other oils solidify and are no good for you – especially margarine! Lecithin is good for correct liver function and memory. Dried fruit contain concentrated sources of nutrients and enzymes.

> Avoid margarines if you want to be healthy, they contain oils that solidify and are, therefore, NOT suitable for the human body at all! They are also heavily processed and contain non nutritional products during the manufacturing process.

HERBS – Chamomile, sage (excellent), dandelion, celery seed (acid waste removal), red clover, vitamin C powder only, alfalfa tea (acid waste removal), licorice, senna pods (for constipation),

Summary of foods and acid / alkaline balance;
- √ Most vegetables are alkaline and produce alkaline conditions for the body,
- √ Sugar is alkaline and produces acid conditions for the body,
- √ Meat and animal foods are acid based and produce acid conditions for the body,
- √ Fats are acid based and produce acid conditions for the body,
- √ Minerals are alkaline and acid based and produce some acid and some alkaline conditions for the body.

HEALTHY NOTES:

Lightly steam vegetables only – if you boil them until soft they will not have much nutritional value and *destroy important enzymes*. Steam, grill, or lightly boil. RAW is BEST!

Forget the glycaemic index (GI), strengthen your digestive system and consume low HI (Human Intervention) foods.

For weight rebalancing remember this key point;

"What goes in (in the way of foods),

versus what goes out (in energy output)

You will put on weight if you;
- Consume more calorie enhanced foods
- Exercise less

You will reduce weight if you;
- Consume less calorie foods and MORE of natures natural foods
- Exercise

NEUTRAL FOODS that do not put on extra weight BUT also IMPROVE your health are; fresh fruit and vegetables, especially greens, lettuce, tomatoes, cucumbers, apples, to name a few.

Diet and Personal Health

It is not rocket science to make a huge difference with your health – you have the choice to do a little, or a lot! This book is to give you the information so that you can make better choices with nutrition, etc., the rest is up to you. You can have those take outs or fast food sometimes, but, make sure that **MOST** of the time foods are nutritional for you.

I have included a daily diet plan, the "Low Acid Diet Plan" previous, to be followed as much as possible throughout the week. Summarizing, the diet includes such foods as;
Fresh fruit and vegetables, rice and pasta, etc., nuts, lean white meats, minimal dairy products (use alternatives soy, etc.), minimal coffee, plenty of <u>fresh</u> water, exercise, laughter, love and human compassion for yourself and others!
Remember; Everything in moderation, including moderation itself! Just make sure that most of the time you are eating right. Easy isn't it?

The bottom line is for the intake to be as natural, pure and uncontaminated as possible. Remember, 'What goes in determines what goes out' in the way of energy conversion in the digestion process, and in feeding all the cells of the body with pure foods. Neither is it any good if the food that you consume is loaded with chemicals, preservatives, etc., and then overcooked in the process.

I STRESS THIS POINT! Be aware as much as possible of what you eat, and question the content or cooking process of purchased food as much as you can. Some food manufacturing companies are out there just to make money and not to look after our nutritional needs. So keep this in mind; your body is not a waste dump, it is a highly organised and balanced living thing and, therefore, needs special attention paid to it! Sure, we are resilient and our bodies can cope with a certain amount of imbalance from our nutritional intake, but, be aware your reserves are being depleted – then we start to age more rapidly

Several years ago my father suffered from extreme tiredness during the day even after a restful amount of sleep at night. After many prognoses he was diagnosed as having lead poisoning. This came about from years of working with pesticides on the family orchard. He is now very aware of chemicals, additives and other foreign substances affecting the food we eat and what is in our environment. This is just one example among many out in the 'real' world where we have to be ever watchful with nutrition and diet. Raw and less processed food the better! Wholemeal flour is better nutritionally than white flour as this is highly processed and just about devoid of goodness.

HINT: Grow your own vegetables in a raised garden bed. Consume, no, <u>demand</u> free range eggs.

A misunderstood approach to dieting exists in western societies: The misconception with western style approaches to dieting is to stop eating. This is not the correct way of dealing with weight management. Eat correct proportions of the correct food, (as natural as you can find and preferably uncooked.)

The secret to longevity is a slightly empty stomach! If you eat until you are exactly full then the digestive process is working overtime, and stresses the body's internal balance. If you are careful of what you eat, (pure, balanced, fresh, low in saturated fats, etc.,) then with some simple exercise you can achieve your weight goals. However, that is not the only answer. We have all heard of some magical formula for our nutritional needs, and the balancing ingredient needed is - the mind.
"I knew there was a catch!" I hear you say. What do we have to do then? We need something to motivate us so we can see in advance or some future result or picture we can draw on. What we should be doing is known as; Painting the picture – getting results in advance'.

Develop the mindset to see yourself in the future: Using your mind to positively achieve your desires and maintain them. Focus all your energy into your new approach to yourself and that which you focus is that which you will receive – this is also a profound law of nature as well. Manifest this view and it becomes reality.

What about exercise you ask!

Exercise can be as simple as a session of Yoga, light stretching, a jog, a walk, or something that can increase the blood and lymphatic flow within our bodies. Did you know, a session of Yoga can be nearly as beneficial for you as an aerobics session at the local gym! But remember you do need some sort of exercise regime to assist the body's lymphatic system to operate efficiently. The lymph system is responsible for the removal of waste products from cell metabolization, basically. By efficiently removing waste products this also helps the immune system work efficiently as well.

Often the labels on a food product are not a true indication of what we are eating. We all know a healthy diet is not the only thing to looking after ourselves – it is just one part, yet a major part to consider. White flour contains some chemicals so as to enable shelf life to be achieved. Check what you are eating!

In our lives we can better achieve our goals if we have something that drives us to make the change. Discipline your habits, then reward yourself along the way. Keep in mind the, 'Results in Advance' I mentioned previously, this is the mentality that will set in concrete what you want to achieve and make things happen as planned.

If you wake tired from a good night's sleep then please consider your diet. What you might think is OK for you to eat may not be appropriate for your body type, or for humans full stop! Check the fur on your tongue. (See section on tongue condition in health reference section.)

> The only way to get the full range of nutrients is from natural foods. Over a period of time depleted nutrition will be seen first as increased illnesses, colds, etc. and not feeling well. This will progress to deep seated diseases; cancers, blood and organ diseases that will shorten your life _and_ alter your DNA chain. This is not so much a sign of getting old; this is more to do with fueling the body correctly and assisting the body to build, repair and defend itself.

But, you ask, what foods are good to eat and what foods do I avoid or minimise? If you are unsure what is good / bad for your diet plan, then one way is to apply a simple 'Muscle Test.'

How to test if a food is suitable for your body or not.
Stand, with left arm straight out and perpendicular to the floor. Next, have someone place in your hand, let you smell a particular food or even think about the food. Your partner then tries to gently, but steadily, push your arm down all the while you are resisting against them. A steady, slightly firm downward push as you resist is all you need to see results. Now, if the food is 'acceptable' for body, you will remain strong in the arm. If the food is not conducive for your body, your arm will seem weak. You will know to avoid a food or include it. This is so simple to follow. The other way is to sit down quietly with no distractions and 'ask' your inner self for an answer to the question and pay particular attention to your inner voice.

This is how you might try this;
Find a quiet spot that allows you to relax, totally and without interruptions for several minutes. As you relax you will open up to the potential of the universe for answers. Then, quietly and calmly ask the specific question whilst focusing on your energetic centre of your body, your stomach. The first answer that comes through in the first milliseconds is usually the answer you are looking for. The secret is to take the first answer and NOT to judge or to wait for other answers. take the first one that comes to mind! This process may take several goes to perfect, but once achieved you can use this procedure to answer almost ANY question you wish to ask of the universe, believe me this works. Give yourself a little time to fine tune the procedure and the potential of finding answers to pressing questions in your life will be astounding!

Grow your own vegetables in your own 'Raised garden bed' at home. For here we can better ensure the food we eat is wholesome and grown without chemicals or sprays of some sort. Here, the food generated from your own vegetable garden will have <u>optimum energy value</u> as well as <u>active enzymes</u> which are so important.

In a nutshell what we are looking for from our daily intake of food is;
- an efficient metabolism,
- proper absorption of nutrients,
- and complete removal of wastes from the digestive tract, the kidneys and bladder, <u>and</u> the lymphatic system.

You will not achieve this by consuming excess red meat, processed foods, dairy products and excess fats.
        Plant an acorn and a beautiful oak tree grows,
           plant a cow and it rots in the ground!
Consume foods that have life energy in them. How do we do this?
Please go back over these last few paragraphs because it is too important for us to overlook!

Our bodies are remarkable structures – to say the least! When given high performance fuel and good maintenance, plus a cleaning program, for our internal system, that is easy to follow and understand we can better achieve optimum health.
You want that true health to be able to, say, play with your son or daughter don't you? What you don't want to hear is this; "Sorry Tommy, but I can't play basketball with you my hip is sore and my blood pressure won't allow it, etcetera, etcetera". See how we can choose to have better health?

You service your car regularly, vacuum the house weekly, empty the rubbish bin – but seem to neglect your own bodies. There are simple procedures we can take to alleviate and improve our health now and for the coming future. My wife and I know several people close at heart that suffered from health related problems unnecessarily when the quality of life could have been greatly improved just by following some simple steps – and we all know someone that has a similar situation or potentially life debilitating illness. Offer them some positive health suggestions: With some compassion, love understanding you can suggest good basic advice for their health. If they choose not to heed your advice, then that is their choice, you have tried your best.

Wisdom should be acquired, not rheumatism; understanding, not limitation. If you haven't learnt much about your body and it's life processes you can plead ignorance, I suppose, but you should pay close attention to your 'Temple' - your divine body. Those with guts enough to do something to reverse it will reap the rewards. Think about this;, we receive less than 50% nutrition because of how the food is grown, stored, cooked, processed, etc.

'*Calorie watching*' as it is known, is good, but you must ensure you also receive sufficient nutrients from the foods you consume. Understanding this point will help your diet and the overall health of your body.

<u>Watch the Potassium / Sodium balance in food intake.</u>
Potassium is found mostly in fresh unprocessed foods. Sodium is generally found in high levels in processed, non fresh, stored foods, etc. Ideally, you need more potassium foods and less sodium foods. (This helps the acid balance of the body).

One final comment on diet and personal health comes by the way of an observation made years ago:
While visiting a local farmer's market I noticed a woman approach a fruit stand. She had bags of chips, sugary drinks and sweets, to name but a few, that were stretching the handles of the carry bag. I overheard her say that she had just bought some fairy floss for her daughter and that all she wanted from the fruit stand was two tomatoes and a red capsicum. I don't want to sound like I am judging too much but I bet that most of her (healthy) shopping took place in this manner. We can have the sweets and processed foods in life, however, make sure that most of the time you consume good wholesome foods – remember the 70/30 rule earlier in the book?

Basic Back Care

(Hint – Stretching muscles and relieving tension in the back significantly helps towards a pain free back. This point cannot be over-emphasized)

Our back supports our daily activities more than we care to think. There are some basic stretching techniques that we can employ to relieve tension, congestion and weakness in the muscles, and the joints as well. Caring for the back through regular exercise of the back muscles will help to remove toxins within the muscles and assist in eliminating compression forces on the spine.

One of the main causes of back pain seems to be our constant use of certain muscles in a limited range of movement, this we can see in our daily activities. For example; we walk with a limited range of movement of our legs during the day. This strengthens our legs and muscles – usually within this limited range only. Then, when we are forced to stretch the leg a little further, say in a sporting situation, then the inevitable happens and we tear and injure soft tissue and ligaments.

Handy hints for better backs
- Sit with your lower back against the back of the chair
- Walk with a good posture all the time – form good habits now. Walk as tall as you can; think of your torso detaching from your legs. Your head detaching from your body. (This also gives you self confidence and great respect from your fellow human being – think about it for a moment!)
- If sitting for prolonged periods, stand up and move about every twenty minutes or so, performing light stretches.

How do we improve back pain?

- Stretch your mobilizing muscles (muscles that move us)
- Loosen tight nerves (by gently stretching)
- Mobilize stiff joints (breathe through the slight pain)

- Strengthen stability muscles (muscles that stabilize us, keeping us in a fixed position – when standing or bent forwards)
- Address your diet

Please read this again and think about what you are reading and what it means to you.

The spine can be;

- Normal (series of glides of vertebrae)
- Stiff (joints do not glide)
- Unstable (not held together firmly)

So, unstable joints tend to become more unstable, stiff joints tend to become more stiff, unless you take more care of your back, and implement some exercises to help.! A joint that is stiff or unstable will quickly degenerate, causing pain and / or inflammation.

It is really quite simple; to avoid back pain we must perform some stretching moves regularly to maintain balance and flexibility of our body. Walk, head up, spine flat, tummy tucked in. Lower back pain can also be linked to relationships in your life and can be a sign that things are, 'out of balance'!

They say that lower back pain can be part of your intuitive system and can be a sign of marriage or partnership problems. They say that something may be out of kilter with this area of your life. May be we all could look at our back pain – is it a symptom of, "Pain in the back" relationships?

One final point on back care

Walk tall with a straight back!

1. Your back will thank you as you maintain correct posture and spinal balance.
2. People will respect you if you walk tall, rather than slouched with head craned forward and rounded back. (Think about this for a moment.)

3. You will think with your heart and not your head, (this will help you get positive results in your life as the heart has wisdom and the head can be 'head strong in judging matters!)

    Think about those last two points when you are with a group of people…

Following is a short list of some essential stretches you can perform at home that will greatly assist your body. (Please consult your health professional to ensure these stretches are suitable for your own personal need. Take care to follow the instructions herein and from your health professional.)

NOTE: If you have strong pain, or previous injuries of the back then please seek professional advice as you can further aggravate the problem.

Top six stretches for you to perform at home;

(Word of warning – <u>do not use the same muscles you are stretching to return to start</u>. Use your arms, as in the example below, and push back to the return position.)

1.

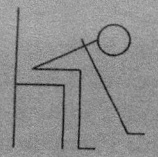

Stretch forward, don't hold your breath, lower yourself by your arms, *lift* yourself by your arms. Support yourself *at all times*

2.

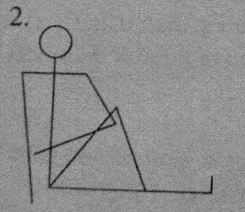

Sciatica – Lift chest, <u>straighten back</u> draw knee to side of chest, movement is to twist torso, breathe normal, hold for several breaths each side. *Shown is right leg bent, with left elbow on outside of knee and head turned to the right.*

3. 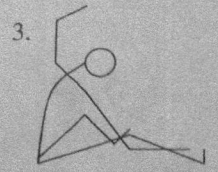 One leg slightly bent, grab foot if you can, elbow pushed up against INSIDE of knee, left foot pressed against right leg, the movement is in the *sideways bend* from the hips and stretches the strong muscles that support the hips and spine – a difficult yet effective move. Repeat for other side.
Note: you are not bending forward, you are bending sideways.

4.

Arms / shoulders on floor, swing leg to floor, alternate each side for 10 repetitions. Hold leg on floor for a few seconds each time to enhance the stretch. Don't forget to breathe!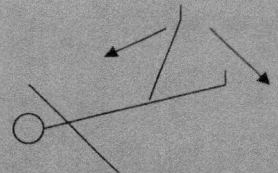

5. 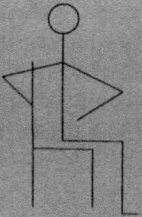 Seated, turn to look over shoulder holding on to seat to assist turn. Hold for several breaths on each side.
Try sitting facing chair back, legs on the side, this will ensure a good stretch.

6. 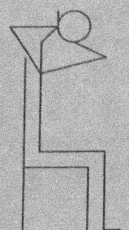 A good stretch of the neck muscles is always needed. Neck muscles tighten and create tension. Stretch forward, when finished rotate head left to right slowly to release any tension left.

Top three stretches if you *can't* find the time;
1. Side stretch of quadratus lumborum. (Ex. 3 above) *This muscle stabilizes the lower spine with the pelvis.*
(This muscle is almost always involved with back soreness.)
2. Supine (lying on back) swing leg from side to side, with head turning in the opposite direction. (Ex. 4 above)
3. *See below* (a) On all fours, (b) slide forward chest to the floor, come up to cobra pose, straight arms if possible, (c) Arch back and return to looking between hands, with back flat and arms stretched forward, head looking to the front.

(a) 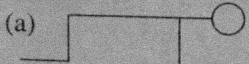   (b)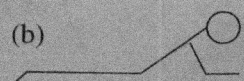

(c)

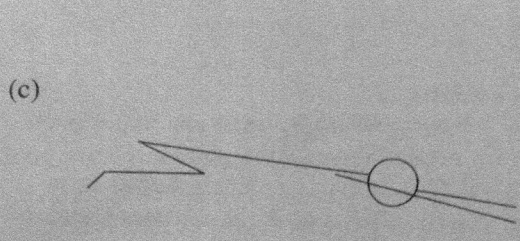

Then finish with the following (Similar to exercise 4 from above);
    Lie on your back, shoulders and arms flat on the floor, knees tucked up, then swing the legs side to side *for several minutes*. Keep shoulders on the floor and alternate turning your head in the opposite direction as you try to touch the floor with your knees. This exercise releases tension in the pelvic and lower spinal region and, I personally, have found this very effective.
With variations you can tuck your knees to your chest to further the stretch effect on the pelvis and spine.
Remember; slow controlled movements – no jerks. *(There are already enough of these in the world!)*

(This also gives you confidence and great respect from your fellow human being – think about it for a moment!)
- If sitting for prolonged periods, stand up and move about every twenty minutes or so, performing light stretches.

The correct technique to improve back pain;
- Stretch your mobilizing muscles (muscles that move us)
- Loosen tight nerves (by gently stretching)
- Mobilise stiff joints (breathe through the slight pain)
- Strengthen stability muscles (muscles that stabilize us, as in keeping you in a fixed position, as when we are standing or bent over forwards)

Unstable joints tend to become more unstable, stiff joints tend to become more stiff.

The spine can be;
- Normal, (series of slides and glides of vertebrae),
- Stiff, (joints do not glide),
- Unstable, (not held together firmly).

A joint that is stiff or unstable will quickly degenerate, causing pain and / or inflammation.

Massage is good for the back muscles and oils such as linseed and wintergreen oils work well to penetrate deep to assist in repair of the problem.

You can lubricate around your joints as well with these oils and wintergreen oil is especially effective as it contains Silica and penetrates deeply to reduce inflammation and swelling.

With stiff backs it generally indicates scar tissue, apart from the obvious lack of exercise.

It is really quite simple; to avoid back pain we must perform some stretching moves regularly to maintain balance and flexibility of our body overall. Chiropractors and Natural Therapists alike endorse exercise.

A point to finish on concerning flexibility of the body;
    As your body becomes more flexible so too your mind!
As you perform these, and other forms of stretching therapy, you will notice not only greater vitality and flexibility, *but also clearer thinking and more creativity.*

Care for your back and enjoy life free of pain!

Section II
Living Happier

(Wellbeing of the mind!)

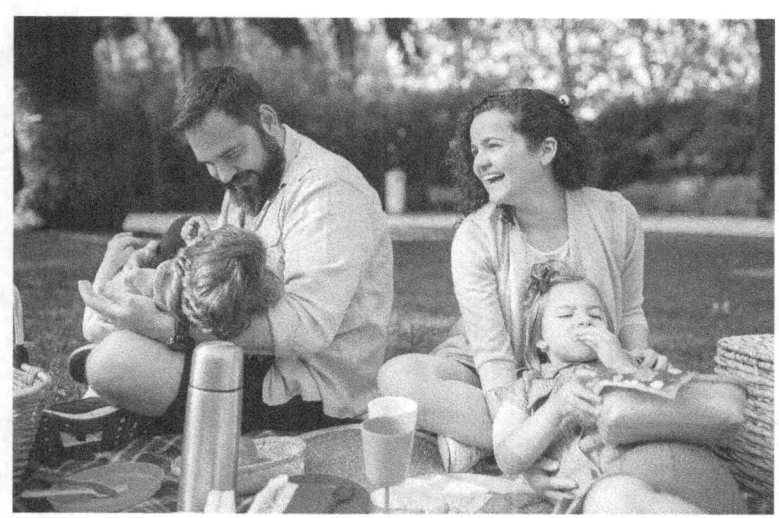

Better relationships?

HINT: Don't put people down! Give out love and kind words, for what goes around comes around!

We often here terms like; "It's the way the world is. We can't do anything about it!" That is a poor compromise in life. From within our own families we can start the impact of our wishes, our dreams for a better world. (Take a minute or two and think about how you come across at home, how you interact with your family and how you feel you contribute to the family, as a whole!) We must overlook those trivial, negative things that we tend to criticize others with and concentrate on the 'big picture' in life. "You left the toothpaste lid off again"! Don't waste time on minor things in life concentrate your positive energies on major things in life – your peace of mind, your happiness and that of those around you!

Can we make a more positive impact on the lives of those around us? Yes, we can! Don't blame the other person, try look at how you come across. Maybe you need to readdress your approach. We can change things by looking at ourselves, firstly, and on a collective basis, we can change the world. To give an analogy here: It is hard to make a U-turn in a cruise ship. However, keep nudging it with smaller boats and it has to change course eventually – it has no choice! You can change things! Nelson Mandela proved this when he stood for his peoples' rights and now the world is a better place for all!

A few pointers to be aware of in any relationship is to aim to spend;

>Major time on major matters
>Minor time on minor matters
>And not the other way around!

Don't dwell on the negative points of a person, it is highly unproductive in any relationship, work on the positive points and you will reap the rewards. If you get uptight if someone, say, leaves the toothpaste lid off then you are concentrating on the minor things in life. This only adds to the negative attitude. There will be people in your life that 'leave toothpaste lids off'. You have to overlook these minor matters and look at the good traits of that person.

Work on your relationships

I cannot emphasize this enough because time goes by unnoticed and soon you will be in the later years wishing you had paid more attention to your relationships with others – especially your own family members. There are some important things to pay attention to, (that you need to master), in any relationship. The two most important needs in any relationship are;
- √ love and
- √ certainty.

People need to know that they can trust your relationship with them that they feel significant, that they feel connected otherwise things become undone. Work hard on your relationships (family, friends, work colleagues), and set those positive foundations in place for a happier life. Aim to not blame or criticize the other person; be the adult we all should be and find solutions to relationship challenges.

You will not believe how you will feel if you ensure this happens in your life! Relationships can be somewhat similar to fishing; when you hook a fish you don't want to pull too hard on the line and you don't want to ease up too much or you may lose it. Working with people is similar and when you master your people skills you can reel in the big fish in life, (food for thought)! One of the deepest principles in human nature is the need to be appreciated. Show appreciation towards others and you will overcome many obstacles to a genuine relationship.

If you wish to be defiant and not be flexible with others then you are bound to experience further conflicts. At, "logger heads" with another, then this is not very productive. "I could not give a hoot what he/she thinks!" Well there are negative consequences with this attitude. So, what could one do in a situation like this? Well, you could smile, shrug your shoulders and say something like this; "Hey, I know things have been a little unbalanced lately, can we talk over a few things, besides I do value you as a friend, (partner, brother, sister…)". With this approach you will encourage the other person to consider, or readdress matters.

If they do not want to talk then let it go for the time being – there may be other issues that 'time' needs to sought out.

Do not criticize others

Learn not to criticize others, nor condemn or complain. This is a negative attitude and very unproductive. If you recall the last time you were criticized for something then your reaction, generally, and you usually become defensive or resentful against the perpetrator. No one wants to be criticized; offer positive support for the other person, constructive suggestions and you will win them in the long run.

People will do better under approval; this is one of our human necessities of existence if you like. I know there will be times that you need to raise your voice to get someone to take notice (believe me there are some that need this), however, if you want change then you need to do this with approval, supporting them, then offering solutions to resolve things for them.

There is not one rule to fix all and we all know there are people that are very set and inflexible in life. However, you can plant a seed of thought in the minds of these people without upsetting them.

If you wish to be defiant

If you wish to be defiant and not be flexible with others then you are bound to experience conflicts in your relationships with others. If you are at, "logger heads", with another; this is not very productive for either person. "I could not give a hoot what he/she thinks!" Well there will be consequences if you take an attitude like this: Wouldn't it be better to be in harmony with others than be against them—you will experience difficulties in relationships, as mentioned?

Don't be afraid to smile and ask where you go wrong.

Not all situations will warrant this approach, however, you will not believe how this will swing uncomfortable situations around – believe me! Communication is a major player in relationships so take the adult stance and discuss things that are on your mind or that trouble you or could worry you in the future.

Why not start at home today!

Three things that can destroy relationships (Poison arrows)
- Poor communication
- Dis-respect
- Gossip

One needs to correctly convey your message to others through better communication, this seems to be at the centre of many relationships, <u>especially family and friends.</u>

There is no room for dis-respect in any relationship – there is no excuse. Showing resect is also a sign of maturity.

Gossip, especially negative talk behind someone's back is poison. You can offer positive support if discussing another person rather than running them down – this is not productive and you will face the consequences of this immature, insecure approach.

Think about how you come across to people you meet – <u>family especially</u>!

Guiding Children

(Hint: Be an adult not a parent with your children—you will obtain better results in the long term.)

True love and care for children is expressed by; guiding their development and helping them to realize their potential through free exercise of their own abilities and aspirations, whether or not it conforms to the parents' ideals. Wow, that's an interesting comment! Staring with our own children we can set about changing the direction of society on a large scale – *yes we can do it!*

However, children still need to know the boundaries in which to function as a balanced human being.

Choices

Giving children choices and decision-making skills is essential for a balanced person into adulthood. A simple example could be; "Johnny, if you clean up your room you can watch that movie on Saturday night you wanted to watch." The child has to make a decision and it is their decision that determines the consequence. Treat them like mature people and they will respond likewise. Another point to be aware of is that if you do too much for your child you will be diminishing their motivation to achieve. Children will respond better if there are clearly defined boundaries. They will weigh up choices and options and become more responsible for their decisions and ultimately their actions. As a parent keep calm and show balanced emotions and you will be able to work more positively with them.

Showing anger around children

Parents should never show extreme anger toward their children, nor anyone else in their presence.

As a matter of fact, yelling at another over some matter of concern is a *sure sign of your immaturity, and probably your inner insecurity of the situation, abilities and capabilities.* Hmmm…

A faulty attitude in children can indicate that the way of life that the parents have arranged for their children is seriously unbalanced. Denial is not good! Make sure you work on bringing up children in a proper manner. Make sure your children receive love and attention and do not show favoritism in any situation – it shows!

Consider what is out of balance with your relationship with your child – and fix it, with love in your heart! Also, being over-controlling can have detrimental effects on children. This may lead to eating disorders in the future – Bulimia, Anorexia Nervosa and others. Eating disorders may be the only thing that the child has some control over. If you constantly badger them then the only thing they can have some control over in the future is eating.

Starting with your own children we can set about changing the world: It is hard to make a 'U-turn' in a cruise ship, but keep nudging it with smaller boats and it has to change course, it has no choice! Life is somewhat similar to a large cruise ship – keep nudging and eventually things will change for the better. Keep in mind also, that goal setting at an early age sets foundations for later on in life as well. Young children need this guidance.

Having trouble with children, (especially teenagers), then look carefully at the home environment, (especially mum and dad), and how they react within the family relationship. There is a lot centred around mum and dad and how they interact with the children: Often children "play up" because they lack love and guidance or direction from one or both parents. Often if the child is not receiving love or in a caring relationship with their parents, they may seek gratification elsewhere in other forms. They may seek affection elsewhere; become involved in drugs. Children need to know what the boundaries are in life and if the parents are not firm then the child may test this out. Try this technique: Rather than saying to your child, "where have you been all night?" Try and be interested in their life and what is going on, then they will often open up to you. I do believe that in dangerous situations you, as a parent, need to take charge that is obvious. Just pay attention to how you come across and try to remember how you felt when you were that age.

It is what you do with your own children at home that has such a profound influence on child wellbeing. Spend quality time with each child, discuss their inner thoughts and feelings before a situation arises.

Communication

Four worlds of communication we all should be paying close attention to are;
1. Self
2. Family
3. Work
4. Community

Self – Communicate with your inner self, being honest and maintaining moral and ethical boundaries makes the process a whole lot easier. You cannot communicate effectively with others if you cannot honestly communicate with yourself.

Family – At least once a week or once a month get in touch with your family in some way. A letter a phone call a visit, keep them dear to your heart. Your immediate family – Of course your immediate family takes priority and great attention. Work with your children don't push them aside when they ask a question. Remember, an inquisitive mind is an intelligent, active mind so encourage them to let their creative side bloom.

Work – Efficient communication here will make work pleasant and pleasing to say the least. Do not hold grudges in the work place. It is more productive to be pleasant and kind hearted – it will come back on you in the future I assure you. I have seen a lack of communication in the workplace be a hinderance in effective business activities. At work ensure you encourage and support your fellow colleagues, rather than criticize and run the person down. Remember, *you get what you give out*, so be positive.

Community – at least be aware of your local community in some way. You may want to give time to some worthy project, etc.

An example of better communication

I would like to give you an example of a situation that happened to my family many years ago whilst camping on one of our rivers.

We had arrived late in the day after travelling many hours and were a little weary and tired. My wife and I started to set up camp while our two boys went off to explore the river. The children came back and after several minutes we heard a raised voice coming from down the river. Out appeared a man who obviously had been drinking and was yelling about rubbish floating in the river that our two children had thrown in there. Now, it turned out that they hadn't thrown it in; it just happened to float by at that time. He was getting very agitated by now and I knew not to continue a defensive tact so I switched things around. I agreed that the rubbish does not add to the beautiful environment and then went on to talk about the fishing to be had here. The man became side tracked and interested in the fishing that he ended up leaving a happy person and wishing we have a great stay on the river.

The point of this is that you can work on improving your communication with others and, using some reverse psychology, can aim for a positive outcome. Try this next time you are in a heated situation and swing things around. Not everyone is nasty – looking for the good in someone is a lot more productive in life!

You benefit from this and so do others!

Control and Power

(Hint – If you don't stand for something, you will fall for anything!.)

There are some out there that love to control others, so if you don't stand up for something then you will fall victim to what their beliefs are, and we are not always right all of the time it just becomes our opinion. You will be better respected if you stand for something – I will leave that thought for you to ponder. We see the results of control and power in everyday life, but tend to accept certain situations. Yes, there are things we can do and steps to take. We may not always get the result we are looking for, however, the attention has been brought to the matter of concern. Let me give you an example;

Your bank has just increased the fees and charges on your account, (of course without consulting you), and yet the large businesses do not receive the increase. Make a noise in some way. Stand up and voice your concern. If you do not want to approach the bank manager directly, then speak to the banking ombudsman, or local member of parliament, or anyone else so the concern you have is aired.

Be astutely aware of the content of media reports, in general. Sometimes the truth is contorted so the subject then becomes sensationalized and receives more notoriety and more sales. In the end we are all equal. This hierarchical thing we have created for ourselves basically by those who hunger for power, control and manipulation of others. "Do unto others as you would have them do unto you". Please do not forget that no one is inferior or superior to you no matter what others tell you. We must never assume anything different, as we are all unique in our own way. I know I am going over something already covered but I must make this point absolutely clear.

Those that hunger for power and control of others are the real losers of society and will fall by the wayside eventually. Take Adolph Hitler, he was a distinctive example of "What's in it for me"? (WIIFM).

This person actually had extremely low self-esteem. Those that make the most noise and yearn for the most attention are actually exposing their inner conflict and desires and 'lack of', traits. We are not inferior to anyone else and, therefore, have a specific purpose for being here. Everyone has a given purpose and once you've found yours then pursue this with all the love, vigour and intention you can muster from yourself. Do not forget this!

Be prepared for the incredible that lies ahead of you in your life pursuits. "Seek and you shall receive," they say.

Keeping Ourselves on Track

(Hint: offer constructive comment – not destructive criticism.)

The news on our media: Only listen to relevant news that could help us all.

We do not need to know about the deaths, etc. that are far and distant from what is important for us.

Are we supposed to be sorrowful and depressed all day just because there was a crime in another country? We are being programmed in a way that keeps us feeling we should be concerned with this negative and destructive aspect.

Turn the television on to another channel at least until that sad and unnecessarily depressing story has finished. We have enough situations to deal with in our own lives without being 'involved' in another negative and depressing situation. Enough!

Forgive and forget and move on and do not hold on to past mistakes as we all make them from time to time. If we know we have made a mistake and hurt others, we <u>must</u> amend it by apologizing or explaining our motives, otherwise we can tend to carry with us, likened to a chip on the shoulder, an issue that will be on our minds in the future.

Choose to only do what brings you joy and if you can't find a way to enjoy what you are doing, then let go and be at peace with yourself. Look inside your heart, for this will be the return to yourself – your true self!

Keep in mind we should be aiming to keep in harmony with the divine order that shapes the entire universe. Look for the beauty in nature as manifested by God (ourselves),and accepting imperfections in our attempt to reshape nature. How do we see ourselves? Imagine looking at ourselves through other people's eyes. What would you be thinking or better yet, what would you rather them to think? "He/she looks to be confident", or "He/she looks to be nervous". I know we should not be putting great emphasis on appearance or looks or mannerisms, however, if you want to keep yourself on track then take a few minutes to really think this point over.

Hint: Only give out to the world, especially your children, what you would like to receive yourself.

Holding onto hurtful situations.

We have all experienced this at some time in our lives: Someone has said something against us in a conversation with someone else, or a so called friend won't talk to you because of ….. well whatever, you know the sort of thing. What do you do about it?

Well, if like most of us, we tend to <u>try</u> and forget the hurtful situation thinking this is the best solution. Sometimes, however, it may be appropriate to question this person as to the reason why they treat you indifferently to others. It may be time to, 'kick over tables', and question matters at hand. .Sometimes we do have to stand up for ourselves, for heaven sake welcome to the real world.

Yelling at another person over some matter or concern is a **sure sign of immaturity and probably your inner insecurity of the situation, abilities and capabilities!**

Wow what a tough statement, (I have mentioned this before). I know there are times when we need to be vocal, however, we do not need to attack the person directly, rather, attack the problem. There is a difference!

Don't hold it in as this may manifest into something that affects you and we don't want this. Don't hold onto the hurtful situation clear the air with this person and put them on track because after you have aired the problem then they will respect you as a human being and you will have got a load off your chest. Am I ringing any bells here?

They probably have many underlying problems that they are projecting onto anyone that may be vulnerable or near them at the time. If these people who dish out these hurtful comments only took the time to look within and analyze the situation and needless hatred and resentfulness resulting form their actions. After all, we as a collective are here to get along with each other as best as possible and not to hold onto the negatives we can create for ourselves.

We don't tell ourselves nearly enough how wonderful we are. We would rather criticize; this is not good and unproductive for us. Do not judge yourself – we are all here for different reasons.

Getting ahead in the world

(Hint: Get your thoughts down on paper)

Get yourself a journal and take notes of things of interest that you pick up each day. If you don't jot them down you can quickly forget them. When you have your thoughts on paper you can 'see' things more clearly – I personally, can say this makes a huge difference.

To help you get ahead in life aim at not comparing yourself with others. We are all here for different reasons so comparing yourself with another is only going to hold you back and this will become a negative thought process that will hinder your progress more than likely. Work on yourself and become that unique individual with unique talents and skills.

If you want change in your life you cannot expect this change to take place if you keep doing the same thing over and over again. If you are not getting the results you desire then; fix things, change things until you see a shift take place.

Problem Solving

If you need to solve a problem try the following;
1. What can I read or source myself?
2. Who can I speak to that can offer advice applicable to my situation?

Speak with those that can offer unbiased viewpoints only, especially matters of the heart.

Unsure what to do in your working life?
First of all, look at your interests, your skills and talents and see what can be linked up with as far as a career opportunity goes.
Ask yourself what you need to do to create an income from those activities or hobbies that can support you and may offer a path into your future career. Once you take this first initial step then you will be surprised how things open up for you. However, if you keep coming up against a brick wall, and seem to be struggling to find solutions then this path may not be the suitable one at this point in time – move on!

Through research into people's career motivations I find that; 'your talents that you have and the events that have influenced you so far bear fully on your life goals and dreams.'

Organs of the body and related emotions.

I have included this information as it is relevant with how you feel inside and outside. Our body's physiological and psychological bodies are linked; many Eastern groups understand this better than Western people, generally. For example; if someone was always angry and bad tempered they would treat the liver. Next time you see someone that is angry tell them they may need to have their liver seen to – only kidding, but you get the picture.

LIVER;
>healthy conditions seen as patience and endurance. Unhealthy conditions seen as short temper and anger.

LUNG and LARGE INTESTINE;
>Healthy conditions seen as happiness, security and wholeness. Unhealthy conditions seen as depression, melancholy and sadness.

KIDNEYS and BLADDER;
>Healthy conditions seen as confidence, inspiration and courage. Unhealthy conditions seen as hopelessness, fear and lack of self esteem.

SPLEEN and STOMACH;
>Healthy conditions seen as wisdom, understanding and sympathy. Unhealthy conditions seen as criticism, worry and irritability.

HEART and SMALL INTESTINE;
>Healthy conditions seen as humorous, intuitive comprehension and gentleness. Unhealthy conditions seen as excessive excitement, laughter and sympathy.

You can see by the information above that our physiological and psychological bodies are all linked together in some way. I have observed, first hand, these links in everyday life. I have noticed people with an emotional symptom often linked to a physical symptom. To give you an example; an acquaintance I know was always sympathetic with those they met. This person had heart trouble, had a major operation and now has a slightly different approach with others.

Depression

Depression is not a mental illness it is a human response and it is something you can learn from. What depression is showing you is that you haven't been living wisely and there is a need for change in your life. Sometime in most people's lives you may experience depression of some degree – for some it is more acute than for others. Now I do recognize that there can be neurological imbalances within the brain in some cases and drugs can offer assistance, however, I do believe that humans need to be achieving in life, otherwise we may become depressed – this seems to be in our constitution. And it is not always a sentence for life. If you have that positive focus in life then you haven't time to think about the bad things in life: Anxiety takes a back seat when we are distracted by something that is thought and time consuming!

May I give you an example;
Let us just say you are a passenger in a school bus that is full of school children. The bus is enroute dropping off children and suddenly, on a down hill run the bus driver faints. You are sitting back a few rows from the drivers' seat and you are the only one that can save the bus from the inevitable. You jump into the drivers seat, take control of the bus and bring it to a safe stop, saving all on board.
This action required you to refocus your thoughts and actions onto more important thing s in life.
Getting you out of the routine of downward, negative thought patterns to focusing on the better outcome of saving the bus. You were so focused on something else.

If you feel a little down at times try to make your life busy. Work on finding interesting positive things in your life or future career, or future relationship. You may want to seek help in some way. Taking this approach keeps you from dropping back into the negative thought patterns and you will find things will pick up even in small positive steps.
If you make depression your only choice in responding to a situation, you are not going to solve any situation. My father-in-law has always

said, "work never hurt anyone," and one key point is to keep yourself busy in life so your focus is on the positive points in life..
Remedy

Get yourself busy in life pursuing your goals and interests. Get help, (professional help), if you can't resolve your situation in a reasonable amount of time. Remember, that you are a unique individual with unique abilities and do not judge yourself against others – this is so crucial to your personal well being and balanced psychological state and future life achievements.

I will make a personal comment here: Some people in life have an easier start, may find success early. I feel they may not be able to handle the more demanding rigors of life as others can; others have that innate ability to persevere with the more difficult challenges in the future and are just being made ready to confront them. (This is just a personal comment so don't read too much into it). Work on your interests in life; find what drives you to do something positive with your time; find what makes you happy in life!

Relaxation and Music

Something we don't do enough these days is take some time out from life for relaxation. Deep relaxation, including meditation, has profound benefits that also help heal the physical body. I find using music helps me greatly. Find a suitable style of music to sit back and relax with, try; classical, easy-listening, world music, or whatever you feel comfortable with. Resist the temptation to use fast paced, heavy style of music – for obvious reasons. For me a didgeridoo and chill-out music works best.

What advantages does relaxation have for your health?
- Clarification of a problem. When you truly relax you can often find solutions to pressing problems in life. When you remove yourself from the daily grind you can open up your mind to receive ideas; to help clarify a thought, or many other possibilities of solving problems can be presented.
- Stress reduction. We all know the benefits of reducing unnecessary stress in our life.
- Improvements in our relationships.

This last point is invaluable for our happiness! While we are in a relaxed state we often go over recent interactions with others, relationships that is, and it is here we can put forward positive light into understanding why we may have acted, or reacted, in a certain way to a given situation. If you think about this for a moment we all could do with some time out to consider the way we communicate with others, especially in times of tension, hmmm…!

Try this; next time you find yourself in a heated argument with someone stop and say to them, "I think I need some relaxation time out about now!" I am only kidding, however, you can see the point I am trying to make and we all could do with some time-out in life. We must try and maintain our adult state in life and not fall back into the child state that can be so destructive in our relationships with others.

Hint: Relaxation can become a key ingredient to your long-term happiness!

REFERENCES:

Carper Jean, *Food Your Miracle Cure*, Pocket Books Simon & Schuster
Carper, Jean . *Food Your Miracle Medicine* 1994 by Simon & Schuster
Editors of prevention, *Healing with Vitamin,s* by Hinkler Books,
Florence T and R. Setright R, *The Handbook of Preventive Medicine* Kingsclear Books
Habibi Soroush M.D *Nutritional Healing* 2001, Habibi Health Resources
Harold, Edmund *Know yourself Heal yourself*
Kloss Jethro, *Back to Eden* by Back to Eden publishing company
Koch Manfred, *Laugh with Health* 1996, Merino Lithographics
Kushi Michio, *The Book of Macrobiotics*
Murray Michael N.D. and Joseph Pizzorno N.D., *Encyclopedia of Natural Medicine* by Little Brown and company
Null Gary PhD *Power Aging* by, Bottom Line Books
Ohashi, *Reading the Body* by, Penguin Books
Reader's Digest, *The Healing Power of Vitamins, Minerals and Herbs*

Information was also sourced from various medical journals and other sources and through personal research, experiences and observations over several decades.

Summary

(Hint: A person who is sick should reflect deeply!)

Health is quite simple, when we truly take full responsibility of our lives and are better informed we can understand what basics we need to pay attention to.

Avoiding the need to take care of our health is not the way of the future.

Sick people don't need candy and flowers; they need our deep concern and warm care to guide them to the proper understanding of why they are suffering.

Look carefully at your life and see how you may have felt when you came down with the illness.

My own personal experience:

Many years ago, whilst working as a door-to-door salesman, I became very stressed and developed pneumonia. I felt I couldn't breathe as I came down with this acute condition. Recovering in hospital, I reflected on my working life and came to the 'brutal truth' that I was in the wrong career. I kept saying, "I will be OK, I just need to get another sale!"

Well, after that health scare I, reluctantly, changed career paths and took on the task of trying to better understand health and what can be done about improving or maintaining it.

Sicknesses, we find, are a warning sign telling us that our way of life has been in disharmony – something is out of balance.

When you came down with an illness in the past think back and take a careful look at what was going on in your life at that time. Was there extra stress, or distress? Were you going through a change of career, or family issues that seemed to overwhelm you? We have all heard the saying about stress leading to stomach ulcers, and this can be true: The body, during the time of negative stress, is releasing more chemicals which can irritate the stomach lining, and other organs as well!

Taking tablets and medicines for the common cold is not the way of the future. There have been some wonderful advancements in medicine, this I agree, however, we can look at nutrition and lifestyle factors more directly to help our long-term health.

A point to remember

Work on your people skills; aim to see the good in people and not the bad.
What approach should we take?
At home, "you left the top off the toothpaste again, that annoys me!" Rather, we should be looking at developing the abilities to ignore the minor things in life that 'annoy' us and concentrate on major things in our relationships with others.

If you attack someone verbally, then their self-esteem is compromised. Better to have a win-win outcome and praise the person for the other fantastic things they do and not stew over, say, a toothpaste lid being left off. It does take conscious awareness to see and then to adjust oneself, but, what a difference it makes to your life, and those around you.

Good health, love and peace always!

Conclusion

Our greatest asset in life is our health!
We need some 70 nutrients a day for the 'correct' function of the human body – most foods these days are lucky to contain a few of these. An example of how we don't receive adequate nutrients from foods follows; If a vegetable is growing in soil that is depleted of Selenium, an essential mineral, then the plant will not produce Selenium. So, we consume that vegetable that lacks a key nutrient and powerful antioxidant, and we do not receive the benefits of Selenium for our bodies.

Our bodies are resilient and can exist on lower nutrition for a while. However, it may not be until we get older before we see ill health patterns taking hold, and may be a little late to start looking at changes to the way we live. Nature has a great life support system in place presented in natural foods. With the right knowledge we can help ourselves to maintain, or improve, our Health 4 Ever. You have the choice of taking full responsibility for your health; don't expect the doctors to have a quick fix to a health problem that may have been brewing for years.
Don't blame all health problems on old age!
The key is to maintain optimum nutrition intake <u>and absorption</u> so the body can function at the correct level it was designed for. Consuming poor quality foods will not prolong your life and will add to a congested and taxing system – with illness patterns emerging. Ultimately, we need to aim for;

- a strong digestive system
- a strong immune system
- a proper elimination of waste and toxins and
- **a peaceful and happy heart!**

Centered around this theme of health are; fresh fruit and vegetables, nuts and grains in their most natural state will help to heal our bodies. This is the mainstay of health! As I have mentioned previously, there are tribal groups around the world that do not get our modern day diseases; arthritis, cancers, etc. They do have a more wholesome balanced nutrition plan that supports the body in many ways. This is living proof that we can heal ourselves; that there are things we can do – I personally, experienced this first hand.

Yes, you can make a difference, search and you will find answers to maintaining your health.

Of course you will need to consult with your health professional before undertaking changes to your lifestyle and nutrition, however, think of how healthy you can be with some little changes and understanding of matters of health. If we think we cannot overcome most modern day illnesses then we are kidding ourselves. I have seen, first hand, improvements o the point that they have been eliminated from the body. It can be done–it is not rocket science! I have observed these improvements myself. I have also observed those that elect to ignore; those that elect to go down the same path; those that elect to expect a quick fix pill when the CAUSE is not addressed. A cure for Arthritis is not in a pill it is in **specific lifestyle and nutritional adjustments.**

Put this health information into practice, combined with principles in Section I, "Living Happier", and you will be on your way to a longer, happier, pain free life.

> Please go back over the points in the book, speak with your <u>qualified</u> health practitioner and make it happen.

Final comment
- **Fruits cleanse the body and organs!**
- **Vegetables fortify and repair the body and organs!**
- If you are getting ill then not enough of the above and too much of the wrong foods, (H.I. foods).
- Certain foods (nature's fruit and vegetables, nuts and grains), have specific properties that can address specific health problems.

- It is not old age, rather, health is intrinsically linked with nutrition and deficiencies – even small changes to your diet make a difference!
- Getting old does not mean becoming sicker. The body is resilient and can withstand some poor nutrition, but your health will gradually decline if not addressed!

Remember my 70/30 rule in health and always look for the good in people!
Health 4 Ever

About the Author

Greg has such a profound passion to give us a better understanding about health. He has sourced and researched information on matters of health for many years from many areas of health Leading on from his intense interest in health he decided many years ago to pursue this often misunderstood area of our life! He has qualifications in Oriental Medicine, double Diplomas in Counselling and specialized in Health Counselling through the Medical Register of Australia. He has appeared on the local radio station with a regular segment on health. He currently resides in country Victoria, a state of Australia, with his lovely wife Jacinta and their two children. They both come from a farming background and this has helped in giving a sound understanding of the benefits of good nutrition. We have good reasons for growing as much of our own vegetables as we can.

He hopes you can take some of the thoughts and ideas in this book and use in everyday health situations.

Health 4 Ever

GREG WILSON

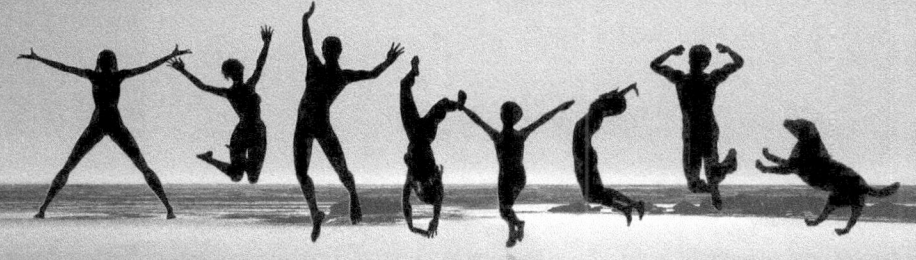

HEALTH
4EVER

www.ingramcontent.com/pod-product-compliance
Lightning Source LLC
LaVergne TN
LVHW021715060526
838200LV00050B/2685